Handbook of Movement Di

CW01023619

Handbook of Movement Disorders

K Ray Chaudhuri
William G Ondo

with contributions from
Kartik Logishetty
Prashanth Reddy
Rosalie Sherman

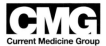
Current Medicine Group

Published by Current Medicine Group, 236 Gray's Inn Road, London, WC1X 8HL, UK

www.currentmedicinegroup.com

© 2009 Current Medicine Group, a part of Springer Science+Business Media
All rights reserved. No part of this publication may be reproduced, stored in a retrieval system or transmitted in any form or by any means electronic, mechanical, photocopying, recording or otherwise without the prior written permission of the copyright holder.

British Library Cataloguing-in-Publication Data.
A catalogue record for this book is available from the British Library.

ISBN 978 1 85873 440 8

Although every effort has been made to ensure that drug doses and other information are presented accurately in this publication, the ultimate responsibility rests with the prescribing physician. Neither the publisher nor the authors can be held responsible for errors or for any consequences arising from the use of the information contained herein. Any product mentioned in this publication should be used in accordance with the prescribing information prepared by the manufacturers. No claims or endorsements are made for any drug or compound at present under clinical investigation.

Commissioning editor: Ian Stoneham
Project editor: Hannah Cole
Designers: Joe Harvey and Taymoor Fouladi
Production: Marina Maher
Printed in Great Britain by Latimer Trend & Company Ltd.

Contents

Author biographies

K Ray Chaudhuri is Consultant Neurologist and Professor in Neurology and Movement Disorders at King's College Hospital NHS foundation Trust, University Hospital Lewisham, King's College London and the Institute of Psychiatry. He is a recognized teacher and active researcher within the King's College London School of Medicine, London, and is the medical director of the National Parkinson Foundation International Centre of Excellence at King's College, London. He also serves as chairman of the RLS:UK group and of the International Parkinson's Disease Non Motor Group, and is a member of the Movement Disorders Society appointments committee and the Task Force on Practice Parameters for PD and RLS. For the Department of Health, UK, he serves on the steering group of the Medicines Management Committee and Gene Therapy Advisory Group, is an advisor of the Health Technology Assessment Committee, and is the lead clinician for the 18 week pathway for management of PD initiative.

Professor Chaudhuri is the author of 172 papers including reviews and book chapters, co-editor of four books on Parkinson's disease and restless legs syndrome (two in press), and has published over 150 peer reviewed abstracts. He has contributed extensively to educational radio and television interviews, newspaper articles and videos. He has also lectured extensively on PD and restless legs syndrome at international meetings in Japan, continental Europe, India and Australia. His major research interests are drug treatment of PD and restless legs syndrome, Parkinsonism in minority ethnic groups within the UK and abroad and sleep problems in PD. In 2005 he was awarded the DSc degree by the University of London and he received his personal Chair in neurology in 2007.

William G Ondo is Professor of Neurology at Baylor College of Medicine, as well as associate director at the Parkinson's Disease Center and Movement Disorders Clinic in Houston, Texas. His medical degree was awarded by the Medical College of Virginia (Richmond, Virginia), and he completed an internship at the University of North Carolina Hospital (Chapel Hill, North Carolina) and a neurology residency at Duke University (Durham, North Carolina). In 1995, Professor Ondo undertook a Movement Disorders fellowship with Dr Jankovic and joined the Baylor faculty the following year. Professor Ondo maintains membership in multiple professional associations and research groups, which include the American Neurological Association, the American Academy of Neurology, and multiple study groups. He is also a diplomate of the American

Board of Psychiatry and Neurology. Professor Ondo is interested in all areas of adult and pediatric movement disorder research and has served as primary, treating, and sub-investigator for many research projects involving those disease states. He has authored more than 200 original articles, review articles, and book chapters, and has edited two test books on movement disorders. He has also served on numerous editorial boards, speaker bureaus, study groups, and has lectured widely. His current research interests include Parkinson's disease, restless legs syndrome, tremor and the use of botulinum toxins.

Kartik Logishetty graduated from Imperial College London in surgery and anaesthesia, and is currently completing his medical training at King's College London. He is a clinical research assistant in Parkinson's Disease, particularly focusing on the recognition and treatment of non-motor symptoms, at the National Parkinson Foundation Centre of Excellence at King's College Hospital, London.

Prashanth Reddy is a specialist registrar working at University Hospital Lewisham, London, and has been working as a specialist registrar in the field of movement disorders for the past three years. He has published a number of book chapters and other publications and is currently pursuing a research degree supervised by Professor Chaudhuri at King's College Hospital, London. He is a part of the Parkinson's Disease Non-Motor Group at the National Parkinson Foundation Centre of Excellence at King's College Hospital, London.

Rosalie Sherman graduated from Cambridge University in medical sciences. She is currently pursuing a career in medicine with a special interest in neurology and movement disorders and is currently actively involved in research as part of the Parkinson's Disease Non-Motor Group at the NPF Centre of Excellence at King's College Hospital, London.

Preface

Movement disorders are a complex group of disorders spanning all aspects of neurological illnesses and range from conditions characterized by too little movement (hypokinesis) to those where movement is excessive (hyperkinesis). The classic example would be Parkinson's disease, while other movement-related problems, such as tremor, chorea, dystonia, myoclonus, hemiballism and tics, occur in a range of inherited, drug-induced and sporadic disorders. Genetics plays an important part in the genesis of several conditions characterized by various movement disorders, such as Huntington's disease, dystonic conditions and myoclonus. Somatization from psychologically determined conditions can also manifest as movement disorders. Finally, sleep may be affected by movement disorders and a typical example would be restless legs syndrome.

To non-experts, movement disorders may appear to be complex, sometimes bizarre and difficult to manage. Diagnosis is based mostly on observation and examination rather than radiology and serological assessments. This comprehensive handbook deals with all the above movement disorders in a holistic manner, providing a detailed "snapshot" view of these complex disorders. As well as being useful to the general physician working in clinical settings where movement disorders often first present, such as accident and emergency departments or in primary care, we hope that the up-to-date information will be useful for trainees and experts in the field of movement disorders.

Chapter 1

Parkinson's disease

Kartik Logishetty and K Ray Chaudhuri

Introduction

Parkinson's disease was first described by the London physician, James Parkinson, in 1817 and later named after him by Charcot. Parkinson's disease is one of the most important disabling illnesses of later life. The characteristic tremor, posture and clinical course were first depicted by James Parkinson in his essay *The Shaking Palsy* in 1817; our description today has added rigidity and bradykinesia to the list of primary symptoms. The modern concept of Parkinson's disease also includes a range of nonmotor symptoms (NMS), some of which (eg, olfactory deficit) could pre-date the motor diagnosis by 1–5 years [1].

Epidemiology, incidence, and prevalence

Currently, there is no "in-life" marker for idiopathic Parkinson's disease and estimates of prevalence and incidence are somewhat inexact. It is estimated to affect 1% of 70 year olds, but it is also seen in younger people, with 10% of cases occurring before the age of 50 [2,3]. Estimates of the annual incidence of Parkinson's disease are in the range of 4–20 per 100,000 individuals. A widely accepted figure for the prevalence of Parkinson's disease is approximately 200 per 100,000 population. In the UK, there are approximately 120,000–130,000 diagnosed cases, but there may be many more that remain undiagnosed. In the USA, it is estimated that between 750,000 and 1.5 million people have the condition [2,4]. Both the incidence and prevalence of Parkinson's disease increase with age, and the prevalence may be as high as 1 in 50 for patients over the age of 80 years. Men are 1.5 times more likely than women to develop the condition. Hospital-based studies have suggested that Parkinson's disease is less common in the Black population, although this observation remains controversial.

Risk factors

In spite of considerable research, it remains difficult to identify the population at risk for Parkinson's disease. The aging process can accelerate the development of Parkinson's disease but is not solely responsible, as some patients develop the disease early in life [5]. Furthermore, the pattern of dopamine cell loss in normal aging differs from that in Parkinson's disease. Certain personality traits and environmental factors may increase the risk of Parkinson's disease but the evidence for this is not robust. People with a family history of Parkinson's disease, particularly in first-degree relatives, are also at higher risk of developing the disease.

It has been postulated that people may be affected differently by a combination of genetic and environmental factors. 1-Methyl-4-phenyl-1,2,3,6-tetrahydropyridine (MPTP), accidentally consumed as a heroin contaminant in the USA in the late 1970s and early 1980s, caused an outbreak of levodopa-responsive parkinsonism [3]. This led to the development of MPTP as an experimental agent to cause selective nigrostriatal cell loss in animal models. It has been recently recognized that welders have an increased incidence of parkinsonism, suggesting that manganese is a causative factor. There have been conflicting reports about other environmental agents that may predispose a person to Parkinson's disease (Figure 1.1).

Genetic factors

Individuals with a positive family history have twice the risk of developing Parkinson's disease, and the risk for siblings is increased significantly if there is an affected sibling with young-onset Parkinson's disease. The risk increases further to 12–24% if both a sibling and a parent are affected.

Mapping and cloning of genes have shown that Parkinson's disease is in fact a heterogeneous group of diseases associated with a spectrum of clinical and pathological changes.

Personality and environmental toxin-based risk factors for Parkinson's disease
Obsessive–compulsive personality disorder
Major depression
Drinking well water
Insecticide/pesticide exposure
Manganese exposure (welding)
MPTP exposure

Figure 1.1 Personality and environmental toxin-based risk factors for Parkinson's disease.
MPTP, 1-methyl-4-phenyl-1,2,3,6-tetrahydropyridine.

In 1996, Polymeropoulos et al. [6] determined that a mutation in the gene coding for the protein α-synuclein (a key component of Lewy bodies) caused an aggressive parkinsonism in a multi-generation Italian–American family; this gene was named *PARK1*. Thirteen genetic loci (denoted *PARK1–13*) have now been implicated in rare forms of Parkinson's disease (Figure 1.2), and at least six of these have been reported to be carried by family members. In addition to "causative" Parkinson's disease genes, analysis has tentatively identified several "susceptibility" loci, including mitochondrial genes coding for proteins involved in the electron transport chain, genes encoding the protein "tau", and *NR4A2*, which is essential for nigral dopaminergic neuron differentiation. *PARK2* (parkin) and *LRRK2* genes are the most prevalent causative genes. *LRRK2* (leucine-rich repeat kinase 2) is part of the family of *ROCO* genes, and encodes for the protein dardarin. *LRRK2* has been associated with both familial and sporadic late-onset Parkinson's disease. G2019S is the most common *LRRK2* substitution, which accounts for 0.5–2% of apparently "sporadic" cases and approximately 5% of familial cases; it is identified more frequently in North African Arabs and Ashkenazi Jews. In the Asian Chinese population the G2385R mutation variant is seen. In Ashkenazi Jews, mutations in the glucocerebrosidase (*GBA*) gene have been reported to confer susceptibility to Parkinson's disease, whereas other studies have reported that 21% of Parkinson's disease patients may carry a *GBA* mutation [7].

Genetic causes of Parkinson's disease

PARK loci	Gene	Chromosome	Form of Parkinson's disease	Origin
PARK1	*SNCA*	4q21	AD	Greece and Italy
PARK2	*PARK2* (parkin)	6q25.2–q27	AR J	Japan
PARK3	Unknown	2p13	AD	Europe
PARK4	*SNCA*	4q21	AD	Iowa
PARK5	*UCHL1*	4p14	AD and idiopathic	Germany
PARK6	*PINK1*	1p35–p36	AR	Italy
PARK7	*PARK7 (DJ1)*	1p36	AR and EO	Europe
PARK8	*LRRK2*	12q12	AD and idiopathic	Japan
PARK9	*ATP13A2*	1p36	Kufor–Rakeb syndrome and EO Parkinson's disease	Jordan, Italy, and Brazil
PARK10	Unknown	1p32	Idiopathic	Iceland
PARK11	*GIGYF2*	2q36–q37	AD and idiopathic	North America
PARK12	Unknown	X	Familial	North America
PARK13	*HTRA2*	2p13	Idiopathic	Germany

Figure 1.2 **Genetic causes of Parkinson's disease.** AD, autosomal dominant; AR, autosomal recessive; EO, early onset; J, juvenile.

Genes underpinning the etiology of the more common sporadic form of Parkinson's disease have been more difficult to localize, although evidence is emerging that mutations in the recessive genes, such as *PARK2* (parkin), *PINK1* and *PARK7* (*DJ1*), and dominant genes, such as *LRRK2*, may play a direct role here too. This is attributed to their capacity to protect dopaminergic cells against insults.

Genetic testing for some Parkinson's disease genes is commercially available but expensive and not routinely performed.

Pathophysiology

The main pathological feature of Parkinson's disease is the degeneration of neuromelanin-containing neurons in the pars compacta of the substantia nigra, which leads to striatal, or more specifically putaminal, degeneration.

It has been suggested that dopaminergic deficiency destabilizes the interaction between the two main functional basal ganglia circuits: the direct D_1-linked (stimulatory) and the indirect D_2-linked (inhibitory) pathways. In Parkinson's disease, dopamine cell degeneration leads to over-excitation of the direct circuit and there is a resultant bradykinesia, which also involves paradoxical excitation of the subthalamic nucleus (STN) and the internal segment of the globus pallidus (GP_i).

Lewy bodies are intracytoplasmic eosinophilic inclusion bodies found in the neurons of the substantia nigra (Figures 1.3 and 1.4). Their formation is a hallmark of dopaminergic cell degeneration in Parkinson's disease. The traditional "top-down" pathophysiological basis of Parkinson's disease has been recently re-explored by the seminal and somewhat controversial work of Heiko Braak [8]. A "bottom-up" phenomenon was suggested, whereby Lewy body formation actually occurs in the brain stem in the lower medulla and the olfactory bundle (stage 1 Parkinson's disease). Lewy bodies are also found in the peripheral nervous system in the gut. In stage 2 more of the dorsal medulla and pons become involved, although it is at stage 3 that the midbrain and the substantia nigra are involved. Therefore, according to this hypothesis, the motor deficit of Parkinson's disease is manifest at stage 3 (Figure 1.5). In support of this observation, several nonmotor features of Parkinson's disease, including olfactory loss, sleep disorders such as rapid eye movement (REM) behavior disorder (RBD), and constipation, which may originate from dysfunction of brain-stem nuclei, can precede the development of motor Parkinson's disease (Figures 1.5 and 1.6). However, the Braak theory cannot explain why some patients with early Parkinson's disease have evidence of mild cognitive impairment or indeed the pathogenesis of dementia with Lewy bodies, in which patients develop early cognitive problems.

Recently, positron emission tomography (PET) of the brain in Parkinson's disease has identified neuro-inflammation in the brain stem, suggesting that the pathological process in Parkinson's disease may be initiated by an inflammatory process within the glial cells.

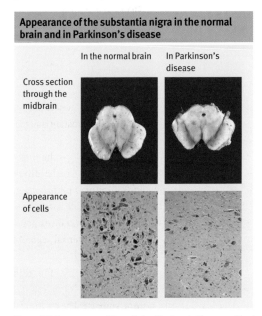

Appearance of the substantia nigra in the normal brain and in Parkinson's disease

Figure 1.3 Appearance of the substantia nigra in the normal brain and in Parkinson's disease. Courtesy of Dr S Al-Sarraj, Dept of Clinical Neuropathy, King's College Hospital, London.

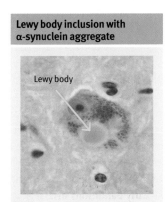

Lewy body inclusion with α-synuclein aggregate

Figure 1.4 Lewy body inclusion with α-synuclein aggregate. Courtesy of Dr S Al-Sarraj, Dept of Clinical Neuropathy, King's College Hospital, London.

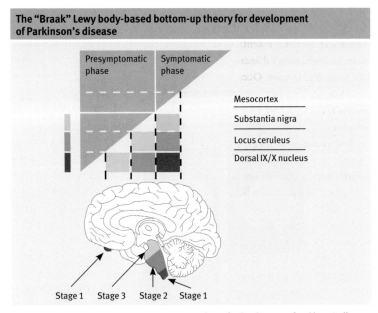

The "Braak" Lewy body-based bottom-up theory for development of Parkinson's disease

Figure 1.5 The "Braak" Lewy body-based bottom-up theory for development of Parkinson's disease.

Nonmotor symptoms suggested as a preclinical (motor) feature in Parkinson's disease

Strong evidence	Suggested links (poor evidence base)
Constipation	Erectile dysfunction
Olfactory deficit	Restless legs syndrome
Rapid eye movement behavior disorder	Apathy
Depression	Fatigue
	Anxiety
	Impaired color vision

Figure 1.6 Nonmotor symptoms suggested as a preclinical (motor) feature in Parkinson's disease.

Symptoms and signs

The motor disorder

Parkinsonism is a clinical syndrome and, typically, when the condition appears to be idiopathic and responsive to levodopa therapy, is referred to as Parkinson's disease. Often the presenting symptom is a slow resting tremor, worse at rest (4–7 Hz) and frequently unilateral. However, 30% of cases do not have a tremor at the onset of the disease.

Tremor often leads both patients and their carers to suspect Parkinson's disease and to self-refer, so it is important to be able to distinguish parkinsonian tremor from essential tremor (ET). Various other forms of tremor occur in Parkinson's disease, including postural tremor, emergent tremor and isometric tremor. Occasionally, a "dystonic" tremor may masquerade as Parkinson's disease tremor, causing an erroneous diagnosis of Parkinson's disease that is discovered only if the patient has a normal striatal dopamine receptor scan.

Bradykinesia/akinesia is a difficulty in initiating, and slowness in executing, movement. It is the most disabling and progressive motor sign of Parkinson's disease and is a core feature for diagnosis of Parkinson's disease using the UK Parkinson's Disease Brain Bank criteria (Figure 1.7). It first affects fine movements, such as fastening buttons and handwriting; the latter becomes progressively smaller (micrographia). Associated movements suffer and one or both arms may no longer swing during walking.

Gait is affected in Parkinson's disease, with patients experiencing difficulty starting walking and taking small steps and shuffling. "Festination" occurs when the patient appears to hurry and then stops suddenly as if rooted to the ground. The face often becomes expressionless (masked face or hypomimia) with reduced blinking. Bradykinetic laryngeal movement leads to quiet, monotonous speech that is low in volume and sometimes repetitive (palilalia).

Rigidity is usually detected on examination and patients tend to complain of muscular stiffness and pain. Parkinsonian rigidity, which can be activated by performing mirror movements in the opposite limb, presents as one of two types:
1. "Lead-pipe" rigidity: a constant resistance to passive movement, in the absence of tremor.
2. "Cogwheel" rigidity: a superimposed clicking resistance like a ratchet, in the presence of tremor.

Diagnosis of parkinsonism (the UK Parkinson's Disease Brain Bank criteria)	
Essential features	**Additional features**
Bradykinesia and two of the following:	Hypomimia ("masked" face)
Tremor (resting)	Freezing episodes
Rigidity (cogwheel or lead-pipe)	(sudden-onset failure of movement)
Postural imbalance, fixed, stooped posture	Seborrhea of the scalp
Gait difficulty (shuffling), short-step gait (with or without festination)	Mental and cognitive disturbance

Figure 1.7 Diagnosis of parkinsonism (the UK Parkinson's Disease Brain Bank criteria).

Useful clinical assessments

Clinical assessment of Parkinson's disease is possible using several validated specific scales and questionnaires. These include the self-rated 30-item nonmotor symptoms questionnaire (NMSQuest), the simple 8-item Parkinson's disease quality-of-life questionnaire (PDQ-8), the motor scale (Unified Parkinson's Disease Rating Scale [UPDRS]) and the nonmotor scale (NMSS). Use of the UPDRS (now revised and available in a new form – the MDS-UPDRS) has been standard, although a more recent addition is the self-completed NMSQuest, which allows patients to declare many NMS of Parkinson's disease that may otherwise never be recognized or declared.

The nonmotor symptom complex

A wide range of NMS is also seen in Parkinson's disease from the early stage (Figure 1.8), all of which are likely to have a major effect on the health-related quality of life of patients. These symptoms include olfactory dysfunction, depression, dementia, sleep disorders, bowel and bladder problems, fatigue, apathy, pain, and autonomic dysfunction.

The nonmotor symptom complex of Parkinson's disease

Neuropsychiatric symptoms
Depression, apathy, anxiety
Anhedonia
Attention deficit
Hallucinations, illusion, delusions
Dementia
Obsessional behavior (usually drug induced)
Repetitive behavior (punding)
Confusion
Delirium (could be drug induced)
Panic attacks

Sleep disorders
Restless legs and periodic limb movements
REM behavior disorder and REM loss of atonia
Non-REM sleep-related movement disorders
Excessive daytime somnolence
Vivid dreaming
Insomnia
Sleep-disordered breathing

Autonomic symptoms
Bladder disturbances
Urgency
Nocturia
Frequency
Sweating
Orthostatic hypotension (OH)
Falls related to OH

Hypersexuality (likely to be drug induced)
Erectile impotence
Dry eyes (xerostomia)

Gastrointestinal symptoms
Dribbling of saliva
Ageusia
Dysphagia/choking
Reflux, vomiting
Nausea
Constipation
Unsatisfactory voiding of bowel
Fecal incontinence

Sensory symptoms
Pain
Paresthesia
Olfactory disturbance

Other symptoms
Fatigue
Diplopia
Blurred vision
Seborrhea
Weight loss
Weight gain (possibly drug induced)

Nonmotor fluctuations
Autonomic
Cognitive
Sensory

Figure 1.8 The nonmotor symptom complex of Parkinson's disease. REM, rapid eye movement.

Confirmation of diagnosis

There are no specific tests for the diagnosis of Parkinson's disease and diagnosis remains clinical [9]. Acute levodopa and apomorphine challenge tests are not encouraged because of high false-positive and false-negative rates.

DaT scanning is single photon emission computed tomography (SPECT) using a labeled cocaine derivative (^{123}I-β-CIT and ^{123}I-FP-CIT); it is recommended and widely used to support diagnosis and differentiate Parkinson's disease from ET. A DaT scan (Figure 1.9) labels the presynaptic dopamine transporter and provides assessment of the presynaptic neurons, which degenerate in Parkinson's disease. ET is likely to show a normal DaT scan, whereas in Parkinson's disease there is diminished uptake of the ligand, usually correlating with the clinically affected side. DaT scan results also appear to correlate closely with the progression of Parkinson's disease. It will, however, not differentiate between Parkinson's disease and other causes of parkinsonism.

More recently, transcranial ultrasonography (Figure 1.11) has been used to reveal characteristic hyperechogenicity of the substantia nigra in patients with early Parkinson's disease. This is possibly suggestive of excessive iron deposition in the substantia nigra, but this technique needs to be validated in large-scale studies before widespread use can be advocated.

DaT scan of the brain in Parkinson's disease

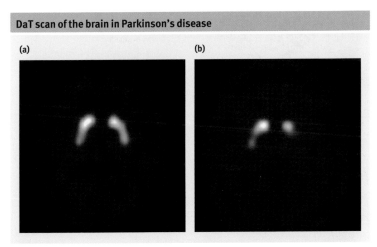

(a) **(b)**

Figure 1.9 DaT scan of the brain in Parkinson's disease. (a) A normal DaT scan showing the comma appearance. (b) DaT Scan in Parkinson's disease showing "dot" appearance on one side, reflecting dopaminergic loss. Positron emission tomography (PET) using ^{18}F-labeled fluorodopa has similar properties and better resolution. It has been used to investigate the activity of aromatic L-amino acid decarboxylase in the striatum and to assess the integrity of the dopaminergic system in vivo (Figure 1.10). However, it is not widely available.

Computed tomography (CT) and magnetic resonance imaging (MRI) are not usually needed for diagnosis, but a brain scan should be performed if parkinsonism is purely unilateral or otherwise atypical, or if additional (pyramidal) signs are present. CT or MRI may also be used to rule out a space-occupying lesion, vascular disease and normal-pressure hydrocephalus.

Diffusion-weighted (DWI) and diffusion tensor (DTI) MRI can be used to aid differentiation between idiopathic Parkinson's disease and parkinsonism resulting from other causes such as multiple system atrophy (MSA).

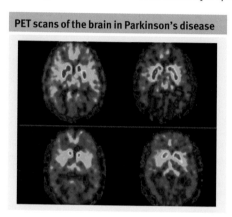

PET scans of the brain in Parkinson's disease

Figure 1.10 **PET scans of the brain in Parkinson's disease.** Upper panel shows normal uptake. Lower panel shows reduced uptake of tracer in the striatum. PET, positron emission tomography.

Transcranial ultrasonography in early Parkinson's disease

Figure 1.11 **Transcranial ultrasonography in early Parkinson's disease.** A transcranial ultrasound of the midbrain showing iron deposition (arrows) of the substantia nigra in Parkinson's disease.

DWI reflects a quantifiable coefficient known as the apparent diffusion coefficient (ADC) and preliminary reports suggest that idiopathic Parkinson's disease has significantly higher regional ADC values compared with MSA. DWI is also thought to differentiate between MSA and progressive supranuclear palsy (PSP).

Management of Parkinson's disease

When to initiate treatment remains a key question and one school of thought recommends starting treatment at the time of diagnosis. The decision to treat may be dictated by the following clinical issues:

- Involvement of dominant hand relative to nondominant hand and effect on employment/occupation
- The particular subtype of Parkinson's disease (bradykinesia-dominant disease may require earlier treatment than tremor-dominant disease)
- The individual sentiments of patients and carers (offer informed choice)
- Presence of NMS such as pain, depression or sleep problems.

For initiating treatment, several guidelines, including the UK National Institute for Health and Clinical Excellence (NICE) guidelines [10], recommend levodopa, dopamine agonists, or monoamine oxidase type B (MAO-B) inhibitors. The development of these medications is shown in Figure 1.12. Drugs for Parkinson's disease work at either the presynaptic site or postsynaptic dopamine receptors (Figure 1.13).

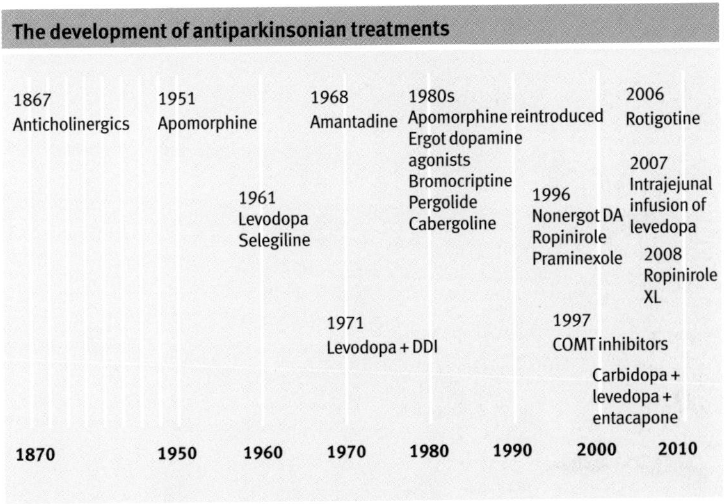

Figure 1.12 The development of antiparkinsonian treatments. COMT, catechol-*O*-methyltransferase; DA, dopamine agonist; DDI, dopa decarboxylase; ER, extended release.

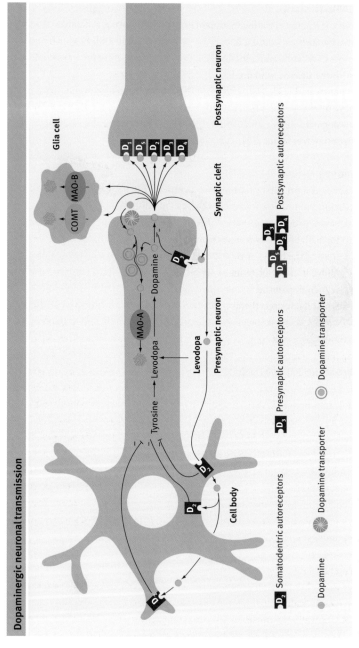

Figure 1.13 Dopaminergic neuronal transmission. COMT, catechol-O-methyltransferase; D, dopamine; MAO, monoamine oxidase.

The PDLIFE study

The argument for initiating treatment of Parkinson's disease at diagnosis is supported by the prospective UK-based multicenter PDLIFE study, which reported a progressive and significant deterioration in the quality of life of patients with Parkinson's disease who are left untreated at diagnosis, compared with those who are treated [11]. The Schapira–Obeso hypothesis also argues for starting treatment at diagnosis because it proposes that, in early Parkinson's disease, physiological compensatory processes are harmful and can be reversed by early initiation of treatment [12].

Levodopa

Levodopa is a precursor to dopamine, converted to dopamine by dopa decarboxylation and restoring the dopamine lost via degeneration of striatonigral cells. Levodopa is usually available combined with a peripheral dopa decarboxylase inhibitor such as carbidopa or benserazide, which inhibits dopa decarboxylase in the rest of the body, or by using drugs such as tolcapone and entacapone, which inhibit catechol-O-methyltransferase (COMT), an enzyme that also breaks down dopamine.

It is best if levodopa therapy is started at the minimum effective dose (usually 50–100 mg/day), in combination with a decarboxylase inhibitor, and given three to four times daily. Dyskinesias and motor fluctuations are a concern. The ELLDOPA study (Early versus Late Levodopa in Parkinson's disease study) evaluated previously untreated patients with Parkinson's disease randomized to three doses (150, 300 or 600 mg) of levodopa or placebo [13]. Levodopa-treated patients showed a significant improvement in motor scores at all three doses compared with those receiving placebo, but the 600 mg/day dose was associated with a dyskinesia rate as high as 17% at 1 year. SPECT suggested an increased rate of decline of striatal β-CIT uptake in the levodopa-treated arm compared with the placebo arm.

Side effects, such as light-headedness or nausea, may be relieved by taking the medication with food or by taking domperidone. Alternatively, side effects can be minimized by increasing the dose of decarboxylase inhibitor. This prevents peripheral degradation of levodopa (and the associated gastrointestinal symptoms) and increases central dopamine concentrations.

Intrajejunal levodopa

In advanced Parkinson's disease refractory to other forms of conventional therapies, intraduodenal/jejunal infusion of levodopa forms an alternate route of administration. A portable infusion pump delivers levodopa in a gel formulation (Duodopa) continuously through a percutaneous endoscopic gastrostomy

(PEG) tube into the duodenum, where it is absorbed and produces a steady plasma level (Figure 1.14). Studies have shown that intrajejunal infusion of levodopa is effective in controlling motor fluctuations in advanced Parkinson's disease, improves motor and nonmotor symptoms, reduces dyskinesias, and allows withdrawal of oral dopaminergic treatment and apomorphine infusion. Quality of life is improved even in patients in whom other therapies have failed. At 6-month follow up a recent international study, with centers in the UK, Germany and Italy, reported a striking improvement in overall NMS burden as measured by the NMSS following Duodopa infusion [14]. Duodopa is licensed in several countries as an "orphan" drug but is not available in the USA.

Location and components of a levodopa intrajejunal infusion system

A   Container of levodopa in a gel formulation
B   Pump
C   Connection
D   Gastric Port, PEG
E   Intestinal tubing

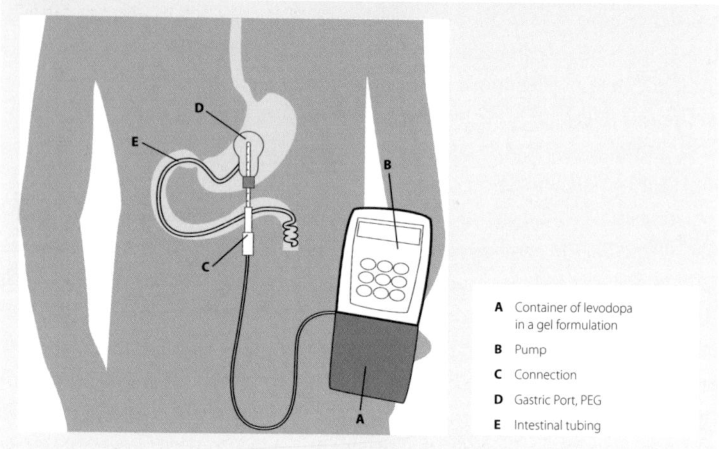

Figure 1.14 Location and components of a levodopa intrajejunal infusion system.

COMT inhibitors

Despite the routine administration of a peripheral dopa decarboxylase inhibitor with levodopa, only 5–10% of each levodopa dose crosses the blood–brain barrier. Much of the rest is metabolized peripherally by COMT. COMT inhibitors, in combination with levodopa and carbidopa, maximize levodopa bioavailability for transport across the blood–brain barrier. Entacapone and tolcapone lead to a 30–50% increase in the levodopa half-life and a 25–100% increase in its concentration-versus-time curve. Although tolcapone was initially associated with several cases of fatal hepatic toxicity, it is now licensed for those who have shown no improvement on entacapone, because it may be more potent. Liver function is monitored throughout the course of the treatment, initially at 2-week

Levodopa-related complications	
Short term	**Long term**
Gastrointestinal Nausea Vomiting Gastritis	**Motor** Fluctuations: "Wearing-off" phenomenon (end-of-dose deterioration) Random "on/off" oscillations, delayed "on" response
Cardiovascular Postural hypotension	Drug-resistant "off" phenomenon (dose failure) Early-morning akinesia, freezing, diphasic dyskinesia Dyskinesia: Peak-dose choreic turning

	Nonmotor ("off"-period-related)
	Pain, akathisia, restless legs, sweating, tachycardia,
	    dyspnea, depression, panic attacks, hyperventilation,
	    screaming
	"Off" period dystonia

	Neuropsychiatric Hallucinations Delirium and paranoid psychosis Hypersexuality
	Sleep related Nightmares Vivid dreams Fragmented sleep

Figure 1.15 Levodopa-related complications.

intervals for the first year. Entacapone with levodopa plus co-careldopa (carbidopa) is also available in a combination form (Stalevo). Meta-analysis of COMT inhibitors demonstrated a reduced "off" time, a reduced levodopa dose, and an improvement in motor impairments and disability, at the expense of increased dopaminergic adverse events such as nausea and dyskinesia [15]. Dyskinesias and wearing off (Figure 1.15) and various other motor complications are usually associated with long-term levodopa treatment, frequently ascribed to a pulsatile mode of delivery. An international study (STRIDE – STalevo Reduction In Dyskinesia Evaluation) was carried out to establish if initiation of treatment with Stalevo at four or more doses a day reduces dyskinesia, but, disappointingly, the results showed it to be less effective than the standard levodopa/carbidopa formulation in delaying the onset of dyskinesia. However, other forms of continuous dopaminergic stimulation are being attempted including once-a-day preparations of dopamine agonists and apomorphine infusions.

Monoamine oxidase type B inhibitors

MAO-B inhibitors, including rasagiline and selegiline, prevent the metabolism of dopamine, thereby increasing its availability in the striatum. MAO-B inhibitors do not cause a reaction after consumption of tyramine-rich foods ("tyramine" or "cheese" reaction) and are therefore safer to use than nonselective inhibitors.

A meta-analysis of 17 randomized trials, examining the effects of the MAO-B inhibitors selegiline, lazabemide and rasagiline on 3525 people, demonstrated improved total, motor and activities of daily living (ADL) UPDRS scores [16]. More importantly, the use of MAO-B significantly reduced the need for levodopa in people with Parkinson's disease. Selegiline and rasagiline can therefore improve motor symptoms and delay the need for levodopa. Although the efficacy of selegiline in treating motor fluctuations is modest, the more potent rasagiline reduces daily "off"-time by up to an hour more than placebo [17].

When MAO-B inhibitors were compared with dopamine agonists, the results suggested that the latter are more effective in delaying the need for levodopa.

Dopamine receptor agonists

Dopamine receptor agonists mimic the effect of dopamine by binding directly with the postsynaptic dopamine receptors. They stimulate dopamine receptors directly and so bypass the degenerating presynaptic nigrostriatal neurons. Five types of dopamine receptors (D_1–D_5) have been identified so far. These are broadly divided into: D_1-like and D_2-like receptors (Figure 1.16):

- D_1-like receptors (D_1 and D_5) – linked to adenylyl cyclase
- D_2-like receptors (D_2, D_3 and D_4) – not linked to adenylyl cyclase.

Improvement in motor function is generally attributed to D_1 and D_2 receptors, which are mostly concentrated in the striatum (caudate nucleus and putamen). D_2 and D_3 receptors are also localized in the limbic regions, which are important for regulation of behavior, mood and emotion.

Ergot-derived dopamine agonists (bromocriptine, cabergoline, lisuride and pergolide) are no longer favored because these have been reported to cause serosal reactions such as pleural, pericardial and peritoneal effusion and/or cardiac valvular fibrosis. Pergolide has been extensively studied and is no longer recommended as a first-line therapy because of the risk of cardiac valvulopathy, possibly linked to 5-hydroxytryptamine type 2B ($5\text{-}HT_{2B}$) receptor agonist action.

The nonergot dopamine agonists (pramipexole, ropinirole, rotigotine and apomorphine) are therefore prescribed in favor of their ergot-derived counterparts. If a patient is started on ergots, renal function tests, erythrocyte sedimentation rate (ESR), chest radiograph and echocardiography must be performed before starting treatment, and annually thereafter.

Of the nonergot dopamine agonists, ropinirole and pramipexole are well-established nonergot dopamine agonists in widespread clinical use in early and advanced Parkinson's disease. Both are effective in early and late disease as monotherapy and adjunctive therapy. Pramipexole, in particular, has been investigated for antidepressant and antianxiety effects, and a recent parallel-group randomized study in people with Parkinson's disease has indicated that pramipexole has antidepressant effects comparable to sertraline. Further double-blind studies are under way.

Rotigotine is the first transdermally delivered nonergot dopamine agonist shown to be effective in early and advanced Parkinson's disease. It delivers continuous dopamine stimulation. Unlike the other nonergot dopamine agonists (except cabergoline), it is effective in a once-daily application. In parkinsonian primate and mouse models, treatment with rotigotine produces virtually no

Pharmacokinetic properties of dopamine receptor agonists

Agonist	Receptor selectivity	Typical dose [mg (mg/day)]
Ergot		
Bromocriptine	$D_1 -$ $D_2 ++$	5–20 (1.25–30)
Lisuride	$D_1 ++$ $D_2 ++++$	1–3 (0.6–5)
Pergolide	$D_1 ++$ $D_2 ++++$ $D_3 ++$	1–3 (0.75–5)
Cabergoline	$D_1 ++$ $D_2 ++++$	2–4 (1–12)
Nonergot		
Ropinirole	$D_2 +++$ $D_3 ++++$	3–18 (1–24)
Pramipexole	$D_2 ++++$ $D_3 ++++$	1.5–4.5 (0.75–6)
Rotigotine patch	$D_1 ++$ $D_2 ++$ $D_3 ++++$ $D_4 ++$ $D_5 +++$	8–16
Ropinirole XL	$D_2 +++$ $D_3 ++++$	12–24
Subcutaneous		
Apomorphine	$D_1 ++++$ $D_2 ++++$	10–80 (3–120)

Figure 1.16 Pharmacokinetic properties of dopamine receptor agonists.

dyskinesias. Recently, the European Medicines Agency recommended that supply and treatment restrictions on the rotigotine patch should be lifted, enabling it to be prescribed to new patients. Ropinirole has been released in a long-acting form (Requip XL), while an extended-release form of pramipexole has had encouraging results in studies and is likely to be released by 2010. Data suggest a beneficial effect of long-acting ropinirole on motor and nonmotor symptoms. Initial data examining the efficacy of pramipexole, rotigotine and ropinirole suggest that they all have beneficial effects on sleep function compared with placebo, as measured by the total Parkinson's disease sleep scale (PDSS) score.

Adverse effects are more common with dopamine agonists than with levodopa. Side effects of dopamine agonists include nausea, vomiting, postural hypotension and hallucinations/psychosis in susceptible individuals or at high doses. More specifically, somnolence or sudden onset of sleep has been linked to nonergot dopamine agonists, but studies have revealed that somnolence can occur with progression of Parkinson's disease and other dopaminergic drugs as well. Patients therefore need to be warned about driving. More recently, behavioral problems such as compulsive gambling, hypersexuality and a complex mixture of impulsive behaviors have been linked to the use of dopaminergic drugs, particularly dopamine agonists. Punding (meaningless repetitive activities) is a particular syndrome often unmasked by dopamine agonists. The exact prevalence is unknown but is suggested to be up to 7% in susceptible individuals (men with early onset Parkinson's disease, history of alcohol misuse or illicit drug use, or affective disorders). Abnormal dopamine release in the nucleus accumbens in response to a reward has been postulated as a possible mechanism. The treatment is complex and requires slow withdrawal of dopamine agonists, use of atypical neuroleptics and/or antidepressants, counseling and input from a neuropsychiatrist.

Apomorphine

Apomorphine is a dopamine agonist that is administered by subcutaneous bolus doses or continuous infusion. People with frequent or sudden "off" periods are suitable for intermittent bolus injections. After the threshold dose is established using inpatient clinical examination and motor rating scales, the patient is trained to use a prefilled apomorphine injection system in which the agreed threshold dose can be dialed up more easily by the patient when in the "off" state. Subcutaneous infusions of apomorphine are appropriate for people with Parkinson's disease who have frequent "off" periods, for whom repeated bolus injections are inappropriate. Apomorphine is administered by a portable syringe driver connected via a butterfly cannula sited in the abdominal wall or subcutaneous tissue of the thighs. The programmable pump delivers 50–120 mg apomorphine over the waking day or the whole 24-hour period. Apomorphine is licensed in the UK and more recently in the USA, but only as injections for "rescue" therapy. Apomorphine infusion also is effective in reversing several NMS with response fluctuations in addition to a beneficial effect on sleep. Nausea and skin nodules may complicate therapy, and the use of domperidone or other antiemetics is essential.

Anticholinergics

Anticholinergics were introduced in the late nineteenth century after Charcot's work with scopolamine (hyoscine). In the mid-twentieth century, selective, centrally active muscarinic receptor antagonists were developed that had fewer peripheral side effects. Anticholinergics block the action of acetylcholine against dopamine within the basal ganglia. These drugs may occasionally be used as an adjunct to levodopa therapy, helping to control rest tremor and dystonia. However, they are not routinely recommended and should be used with great caution in older parkinsonian patients because of the risk of inducing a confusional state and aggravating dementia.

Amantadine

Amantadine was initially investigated as an antiviral agent but was found to be effective in Parkinson's disease by chance, due to its enhancement of dopamine release from presynaptic terminals. There is a paucity of studies documenting the efficacy of amantadine versus placebo or levodopa in the early treatment of Parkinson's disease. The limited data suggest that amantadine relieves tremor in early Parkinson's disease while improving levodopa-induced dyskinesias in later Parkinson's disease. Its primary role is in reduction of dyskinesia [18]. Although amantadine is available for treatment of mild Parkinson's disease symptoms, levodopa and dopamine agonists are more appropriate as a first choice (according to the NICE guidelines).

Neuroprotection

Neuroprotection is a process in which a treatment beneficially affects the underlying pathophysiology of Parkinson's disease. Neuroprotective therapies currently under investigation include caffeine, minocycline, nicotine, estrogen, creatine, lazaroids, bioenergetics, anti-apoptotic drugs (CEP-1347, TCH-346), GM-1 ganglioside and GP_i-1485. MAO-B inhibitors and dopamine agonists have been clinically evaluated for neuroprotective properties with positive results in animal models. However, a number of methodological problems with the studies have prevented their recommendation specifically for neuroprotection, whereas trials with CEP-1347 and TCH 346 have been negative [19]. Delayed start clinical trials have been used and the ADAGIO study with rasagiline suggests a beneficial effect in those started early versus late at 1 mg dose [20]. A similar delayed-start study with pramipexole (the PROUD study) is under way. Coenzyme Q10 has shown encouraging potential as a neuroprotective agent. Mitochondrial complex I activity is reduced in postmortem substantia nigra and in the platelets of people with Parkinson's disease. Coenzyme Q10 is the electron acceptor for complexes I and II and as a result is a potent antioxidant. The level of coenzyme Q10 is reduced in platelet mitochondria in Parkinson's disease. There have been 15 completed clinical trials examining neuroprotection testing 13 different drugs in 18 double-blind studies usually involving patients with early Parkinson's disease, largely relying on motor and nonmotor outcomes [21]. Six of these 13 trials have reported a possible neuroprotective effect.

Stereotactic thalamotomy and deep brain stimulation

Lesioning of the thalamus was shown to reduce contralateral tremor; lesioning of the STN corrected all three cardinal symptoms. It has been demonstrated that surgical ablation of the GP_i significantly reduced dyskinesias (pallidotomy) [22]. The procedure, however, had less of an effect on tremor and rigidity. Left-sided pallidotomy is associated with reduced verbal fluency, although bilateral procedures are associated with dysarthria, dysphonia and gait disturbance.

The hypothesis that deep brain stimulation (DBS) (Figures 1.17 and 1.18) could inhibit tremor and dyskinesias was proposed when it was found that electrical impulses applied during preoperative testing had this effect. The technology was already available from pain pathway stimulation. Alim Benabid's group [23] in France has pioneered this approach in different movement disorders since 1987. DBS can be used to create electrical depolarization of neurons in any basal ganglia site, and DBS of the STN is the currently favored approach and is in worldwide use. Meta-analysis of outcomes from cohorts of patients undergoing DBS of the STN suggest that dyskinesia is reduced by 69.1% (95% confidence interval [CI]: 62.0–76.2%), the daily "off" period is reduced by 68.2% (95% CI: 58–79%) and health-related quality of life is improved by 34.5 ± 15.3%. Most studies have excluded patients over the age of 75 years and the most common serious adverse event is intracranial hemorrhage, reported in 3.9% of patients, and psychiatric sequelae are common. Infection rates have an incidence of 1.6%, and replacement of portions of the device is needed in 4.4% of patients.

Location of a deep brain stimulation device

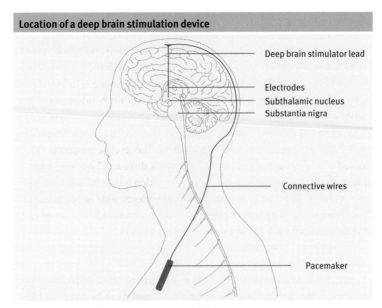

Deep brain stimulator lead

Electrodes
Subthalamic nucleus
Substantia nigra

Connective wires

Pacemaker

Figure 1.17 Location of a deep brain stimulation device.

Appearance of the subcutaneous deep brain stimulation device

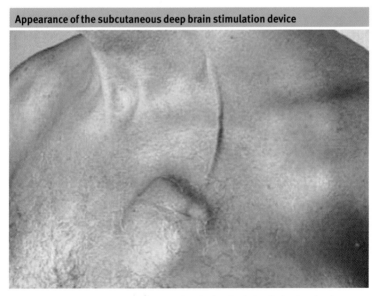

Figure 1.18 Appearance of the subcutaneous deep brain stimulation device. A patient's subcutaneous deep brain stimulation unit is wired through to his subthalamic nucleus.

Other adverse events are dystonia, diplopia, sleepiness, paresthesias, dysarthria, nausea and dysphagia; they occurred considerably more frequently in patients with bilateral implants (52%) than in those with unilateral implants (31%). Economic modeling performed by NICE suggested that bilateral STN DBS costs £19,500 per quality-adjusted life-year (QALY) in comparison to £1998 for standard Parkinson's disease care in the UK. Therefore, bilateral STN stimulation is recommended only for those patients whose symptoms are refractory to the best medical treatment, who are biologically fit with no clinical comorbidity and who have no active mental health problems [24].

Transplant therapies

Neurorestoration refers to increasing the numbers of dopaminergic neurons by techniques such as cell implantation and nerve growth factor infusion. Although there is currently no real surgical alternative to DBS, dopaminergic cell transplant and intraputaminal delivery of glial cell-line-derived neurotropic factor (GDNF) are being investigated as a form of restorative treatment.

A number of possible sources for dopaminergic replacement have been investigated, including autografts of carotid, adrenal medulla and sympathetic ganglion tissue, primary allografts of fetal ventral mesencephalon tissue, and porcine xenografts. Today, investigation is focused on the three types of stem cells: embryonic, neural and mesenchymal. Transplantation in the animal model has proved that it is capable of relieving symptoms and restoring brain function.

Human embryonic stem cells (hESCs) are considered the best candidate stem cell sources for transplantation. They have the unique characteristic of being able to proliferate in an undifferentiated state. They are also able to differentiate into all lineages in vivo and into many cell types in vitro, including neural precursor cells (NPCs). By co-culturing the NPCs with feeder cells that have stromal cell-derived inducing activity, and then using a sequence of differentiation steps (particularly with the fibroblast growth factor FGF-8, sonic hedgehog and ascorbic acid), a significant proportion of the hESCs can adopt a dopaminergic phenotype [25]. When differentiated monkey ESCs were implanted into MPTP-treated monkey striatum, PET at 14 weeks revealed increased fluorodopa uptake and improvement of motor signs.

Subsequent implantation into a rat model of Parkinson's disease, first using hESCs differentiated using stromal mouse cells and more recently with hESCs differentiated using human fetal midbrain astrocytes, showed symptomatic benefit at 8 weeks [26]. The next challenge is in transferring these discoveries into the clinical arena. Although the brain is recognized as an immunologically privileged site, there is an established risk of allograft rejection and teratoma formation.

Although research has largely focused on the use of stem cells, the results of two recently published double-blind placebo-controlled trials using ventral mesencephalon allografts showed disappointing long-term results, including development of disabling graft-induced dyskinesias, the so-called "run away dyskinesias". Recently, three postmortem studies have assessed the long-term effect on fetal transplants in advanced Parkinson's disease and have reported development of Lewy bodies within the transplanted neurons, further underlining the limitation of this approach [27].

Glial-cell-line-derived neurotropic factor

GDNF promotes and supports dopaminergic neuronal cell growth in vitro, and has been shown to have protective effects on dopaminergic neurons in animal models. Kordower et al. [28] reported one patient with a 23-year history of Parkinson's disease who developed side effects after intraventricular infusion of GDNF, with no improvement in parkinsonian symptoms and no evidence of regeneration at postmortem examination. However, an open-label Phase I safety trial in five patients with Parkinson's disease showed improvement in the "off" state and dyskinesias after 1 year, with a 28% increase in putaminal ^{18}F-labeled dopa uptake on PET scans. A subsequent Phase II, double-blind, placebo-controlled study in 34 patients with advanced Parkinson's disease failed to show any clinical benefit. Trials with GDNF have been halted because there is concern that GDNF infusion may cause cerebellar lesions as seen in animal models.

Retinal cell transplantation

Retinal pigment epithelium (RPE) is a source of dopamine. In vitro rat models using a conditioned medium derived from RPE resulted in increased neuritic growth of 78% in striatal neurons, suggesting a potential benefit for RPE transplantation in Parkinson's disease. Spheramine is a cell-based therapy in which normal dopamine-producing cells, such as retinal epithelium, are attached to microcarriers and injected into the basal ganglia.

One small open-label study in six patients, involving unilateral stereotactic putaminal transplantation of RPE cells attached to biocompatible microcarriers, showed a 48% improvement in the primary outcome measure at 12 months [29]. However, a recently completed Phase IIb randomized controlled trial of sham surgery involving RPE failed to show any significant benefit and has thus been discontinued, and the future of RPE remains unclear.

After the apparent failure of this cell-based approach, there has been a switch of focus to gene-based therapies. Of particular interest is ProSavin, which uses a LentiVector delivery system to induce expression of the three enzymes responsible for dopamine production, and thus induce reprogrammed cells to endogenously produce dopamine. A Phase I/II trial is ongoing.

Nondopaminergic drugs for various nonmotor symptoms of Parkinson's disease

Drugs	Class	Condition	Clinical Studies
Paroxetine	SSRI	Depression/anxiety	Phase II
Sertraline	SSRI	Depression/anxiety	Phase IV
Atomoxetine	SSRI and SNRI	Depression/anxiety	Phase IV study underway
Duloxetine	SSRI and SNRI	Depression/anxiety	Phase IV (open-label) study underway
Venlafaxine	SSRI and SNRI	Depression/anxiety	Phase III compared with paroxetine underway
Desipramin	SNRI	Depression/anxiety	Phase IV completed
Pimavanserin (ACP-103)	5-HT$_{2A}$ inverse agonist	Psychosis/visual hallucinations	Phase II completed
Memantine	NMDA receptor antagonist	Cognition	Phase III/IV trials underway
Rivastigmine patch	Cholinesterase inhibitor	Cognition	Phase III
Safinamide	MAO-B inhibitor, dopamine and noradrenaline reuptake inhibitor, Na$^+$/Ca^{2+} channel blocker, glutamate release inhibitor	Cognition	Phase III study underway
Acamprosate (calcium acetyl-homotaurine)	Reduces glutamate-mediated transmission	Behavioral problems (impulse control disorders)	Phase II study underway (for compulsive behaviour and cravings)
Caffeine	Nonspecific adenosine antagonist	Excessive daytime sleepiness	Phase III study underway
BF 2.649	Histamine H$_3$ inverse agonist	Excessive daytime sleepiness	Phase III study underway
L- threo-3,4-dihydroxyphenylserine	An artificial amino acid that is decarboxylated to noradrenaline by aromatic L- amino acid decarboxylase	Orthostatic hypotension	Phase II study completed Phase III study underway
Solifenacin succinate	Muscarinic antagonist	Urge incontinence	Phase IV study

Figure 1.19 Nondopaminergic drugs for various nonmotor symptoms of Parkinson's disease. 5-HT, 5-hydroxytryptamine; MAO, monoamine oxidase; NMDA, N-methyl-D-aspartic acid; SNRI, serotonin norepinephrine reuptake inhibitor; SSRI, selective serotonin reuptake inhibitor.

Nondopaminergic drug therapy

A number of drugs are currently in development (Figure 1.19) that address various NMS of Parkinson's disease.

Specialist nursing care

The role of a specialist nurse in Parkinson's disease is primarily to offer a route of communication for advice and ongoing support. In the UK, over 250 PD nurse specialists now offer invaluable clinical service related to holistic management of PD. The service of PDNS is nationally recognised and forms an integral part of the recommendation for management of PD by NICE in the UK. In particular, services such as apomorphine, duodopa and deep brain stimulation are heavily dependent on management input from the PDNS. An independent assessment of patient satisfaction related to the provision of a specialist nurse demonstrated significant results [30].

Physiotherapy

A physiotherapist is a healthcare professional who emphasizes the use of physical approaches in the promotion, maintenance and restoration of an individual's physical, psychological and social well-being, encompassing variations in health status. Thus in Parkinson's disease, the help of a physiotherapist can maximize the functional capacity of a patient and his or her role within society. Visual or audio gait cueing (stepping over a line or stepping to music) can be very effective for patients with gait freezing.

Occupational therapy

The purpose of occupational therapy is to promote health and well-being through occupation. By enabling people to participate in the activities of daily living, occupational therapists promote independence, safety, confidence, mobility and self-care.

In patients with Parkinson's disease, occupational therapists aim primarily to maintain the interactions of a patient with their family and workplace, and within themselves. The last of these aims specifically addresses the improvement of personal self-care activities (eating, drinking, washing and dressing) and environmental issues to improve safety and motor function.

Speech and language therapy

Impaired speech is a common manifestation of Parkinson's disease that increases in frequency and intensity with disease progression. The "hypokinetic dysarthria" that is characteristic of Parkinson's disease is defined by monotony, decreased amplitude and pitch range, varying rate, and difficulties in speech initiation.

Speech dysfunction in Parkinson's disease is addressed by the Lee Silverman Voice Treatment (LSVT). The program focuses on improving voice loudness with immediate carry over into daily communication. LSVT helps individuals with Parkinson's disease to recognize that their voice is too soft, convince them that a louder voice is within normal limits and makes them comfortable using the new louder voice.

Pacing boards, voice amplifiers, digitized speech output systems, recorded voice messages and microcomputer-based wearable biofeedback devices are alternative options available to the speech and language therapist to treat hypokinetic dysarthria in Parkinson's disease.

Palliative care

The goal of palliative care is achievement of the best quality of life for patients and their families. Falls, fractures, aspiration pneumonia, drooling of saliva, and poor nutrition are all complications that palliative care seeks to prevent.

The "palliative phase" in Parkinson's disease has been defined by the following:
- Inability to tolerate adequate dopaminergic therapy
- Unsuitability for surgery
- The presence of advanced comorbidity.

NICE has produced recommendations for palliative care in Parkinson's disease. Importantly, it must always be provided in the context of the wishes and circumstances of the patient and the family or caregiver. Realistic goals need to be agreed jointly by the patient or family and the multidisciplinary team caring for the patient.

Cost of care

Social services costs account for 38% of total costs of care and tend to increase with increasing age. Total annual direct costs are estimated to be £4189 for patients living at home, £15,355 for patients whose time is divided between home and an institution and £19,338 for patients in full-time institutional care [31]. In later stages of Parkinson's disease there appears to be decreased drug efficacy and an increased sensitivity to unwanted effects of dopaminergic medication, particularly hallucinations. In an effort to balance symptom relief with side effects, withdrawal of dopaminergic drugs is often recommended, and optimization of medication should be closely reviewed.

Mortality and prognosis

The most widely used staging system for Parkinson's disease was defined by Hoehn and Yahr in 1967:
- Stage 1: symptoms on one side of the body
- Stage 2: symptoms on both sides of the body, without balance impairment
- Stage 3: balance impairment, but physically independent

A hypothetical progression pattern of motor and nonmotor features in Parkinson's disease

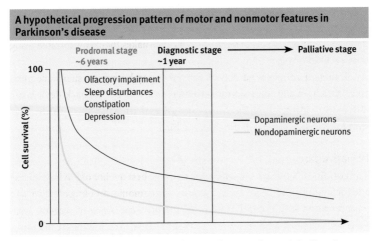

Figure 1.20 A hypothetical progression pattern of motor and nonmotor features in Parkinson's disease. A quartet of nonmotor symptoms may be present before the motor diagnosis becomes apparent.

- Stage 4: severe disability, but still able to walk or stand unassisted
- Stage 5: unable to walk or stand unless assisted.

Alternatively, MacMahon and Thomas have proposed a functional four-stage paradigm that can be used to identify clinical needs, priorities and management plans. Starting with the "diagnostic stage", this model progresses through the "maintenance stage" and the "complex stage," and ends in the "palliative stage".

It is likely that motor and nonmotor progression in Parkinson's disease (Figure 1.20) is nonlinear and NMS may identify a presymptomatic period. It is generally appreciated that there are latencies to Hoehn and Yahr stages 4 or 5 of approximately 7 years, and around 70% of patients are dead or severely disabled by year 10 [32]. However, there is significant heterogeneity in progression rates of Parkinson's disease dependent on etiologically diverse disease entities. For example, patients with early onset Parkinson's disease carrying the parkin mutation are found to have very slowly progressive disease, with latencies in reaching Hoehn and Yahr stages 4 or 5 of up to 40 years.

Overall, the natural history of Parkinson's disease is also associated with an increasing prevalence of NMS, with dementia likely to be inevitable at 20 years, as reported recently [32].

In 1967, Hoehn and Yahr published the first mortality study [33] of Parkinson's disease in the pre-levodopa era and reported that up to 61% of patients were severely disabled or dead after 5–9 years of follow-up, which increased to more than 80% in those followed up for more than 10 years; overall, mortality was three times that expected in the general population. Subsequently, over 20 reports on Parkinson's disease and mortality have been published: two reported a less than 1.5-fold increase in mortality compared with the general population, 11 reported an increase of 1.5–2.0 times, and the others reported rates of more than twice. Disability and mortality in Parkinson's disease appear to show a sex difference, with significantly greater female mortality, although there are other studies suggesting a poorer prognosis in men.

A recent study by Japanese investigators suggested a mean lifespan of 71.9 years for men and 74.2 for women. In Japan, female patients appear to lose approximately 7 years of life compared with men once Parkinson's disease has been diagnosed [34].

Although, with modern treatment, the life expectancy of patients with Parkinson's disease appears to have been prolonged, their lifespan is still probably less than that of the general population, as indicated in the Japanese study. Studies have suggested that relative survival for people with Parkinson's disease diagnosed before the age of 60 is similar to that for the general population, but relative survival is less than expected for those who are older at diagnosis. Pre-levodopa the mortality ratio for Parkinson's disease was 3.0, compared with the general population, and this was reported to have fallen to 1.86 according to the 15-year study by Hely and colleagues from Sydney published in 2005 [35]. However, the same group has now reported a mortality ratio of 3.1 at 20-year follow-up of the same cohort; rates, therefore, appear to be similar to the pre-levodopa era [36]. The confusion about mortality in Parkinson's disease may partly be because the disease itself is not a primary or direct cause of death. A recent 20-year follow-up study in Austria has reported that the survival rate patients who have had Parkinson's disease for up to 10 years is similar to normal control population, while there is a modest rise in mortality in those with a disease duration over 10 years [37]. Male gender, presence of gait disorder and absence of rest tremor appear to predict poorer prognosis. The cause of death in Parkinson's disease is most commonly a secondary comorbid disorder [38]. However, a recent study on PD patients in England and Wales suggests that PD mortality rates are decreasing [39]. It is unclear whether this is due to an increased survival for PD patients, a decline in incidence of PD, or a combination of both.

Conclusions

Parkinson's disease is a multitransmitter deficiency disease that leads to a constellation of motor and nonmotor symptoms. Whilst the primary motor symptoms are well understood, continuing research aims to better characterize NMS, including sleep disorders, neuropsychiatric disorders and autonomic dysfunction.

Occasionally, it may be impossible to distinguish between the wide range of conditions – degenerative, drug-induced, vascular, and metabolic – that may cause a parkinsonian syndrome from true Parkinson's disease. However, advances in our understanding of the natural history and imaging techniques have improved diagnostic accuracy.

Although major advances in drug therapy have been made, we still lack robust disease-modifying therapy. The recent ADAGIO trial with rasagiline, however, has shown some promise regarding neuroprotection. Data soon to be reported from other trials, such as PROUD, may further advance our treatment strategies. Intrajejunal infusion of levodopa and the rotigotine skin patch reflect advances in delivery option of treatment for Parkinson's disease.

Treatment of NMS remains a key unmet need in Parkinson's disease. Robust clinical trials are required so that an adequate evidence base for treatment of NMS of Parkinson's disease can be established. This, in turn, will enhance a holistic approach to patient care and improve quality of life for people with Parkinson's disease and their caregivers.

References

1. Chaudhuri KR, Healy DG , Schapira AH, et al. Non-motor symptoms of Parkinson's disease: diagnosis and management. Lancet Neurol 2006; 5:235–245.
2. De Rijk MC, Tzourio C, Breteler MMB, et al. Prevalence of parkinsonism and Parkinson's disease in Europe: the EUROPARKINSON collaborative study. J Neurol Neurosurg Psychiatry 1997; 62:10–15.
3. Ben-Shlomo Y. How far are we in understanding the cause of Parkinson's disease? J Neurol Neurosurg Psychiatry 1996; 61:4–16.
4. Zhang Z, Roman G. Worldwide occurrence of Parkinson's disease: an updated review. Neuroepidemiology 1993; 12:195–208.
5. Bender A, Krishnan KJ, Morris CM, et al. High levels of mitochondrial 6 DNA deletions in substantia nigra neurons in aging and Parkinson disease. Nat Genet 2006; 38:5151–5157.
6. Polymeropoulos MH, Higgins JJ, Golbe LI, et al. Mapping of a gene for Parkinson's disease to chromosome 4q21-q23. Science 1996; 274:1197–1199.
7. Pankratz N, Foroud T. Genetics of Parkinson disease. Genet Med 2007; 9:801–811.
8. Braak H, Del Tredici K, Rüb U, et al. Staging of brain pathology related to sporadic Parkinson's disease. Neurobiol Aging 2003; 24:197–211.
9. Hughes AJ, Daniel SE, Ben-Shlomo Y, et al. The accuracy of diagnosis of parkinsonian syndromes in a specialist movement disorder service. Brain 2002; 125:861–870.
10. National Institute for Health and Clinical Excellence (NICE). Parkinson's Disease: Diagnosis and management in Primary and Secondary Care, NICE Clinical Guideline 35. London: NICE, 2006. www.nice.org.uk/CG035fullguideline .
11. Grosset D, Taurah L, Burn DJ, et al. A multicentre longitudinal observational study of changes in self reported health status in people with Parkinson's disease left untreated at diagnosis. J Neurol Neurosurg Psychiatry 2007; 78:465–469.

12. Schapira A, Obeso J. Timing of treatment initiation in Parkinson's disease: a need for reappraisal? Ann Neurol 2006; 59:559–565.

13. Parkinson Study Group. Levodopa and the progression of Parkinson's disease. N Engl J Med 2004; 351:2498–2508.

14. Honig H, Antonini A, Martinez-Martin P, et al. Intrajejunal levodopa infusion in Parkinson's disease: a pilot multicenter study of effects on nonmotor symptoms and quality of life. Mov Disord 2009, in press.

15. Deane KH, Spieker S, Clarke CE. Catechol-O-methyltransferase inhibitors for levodopa-induced complications in Parkinson's disease. Cochrane Database Syst Rev 2004; 4:CD004554.

16. Ives NJ, Stowe RL, Marro J, et al. Monoamine oxidase type B inhibitors in early Parkinson's disease: metaanalysis of 17 randomised trials involving 3525 patients. Br Med J 2004; 329:593.

17. The Parkinson Study Group. A randomized placebo-controlled trial of rasagiline in levodopa-treated patients with Parkinson's disease and motor fluctuations. The PRESTO Study. Arch Neurol 2005; 62:241–248.

18. Pahwa R, Factor SA, Lyons KE, et al. Practice parameter: treatment of Parkinson disease with motor fluctuations and dyskinesia (an evidence-based review): report of the Quality Standards Subcommittee of the American Academy of Neurology. Neurology 2006; 66:983–995.

19. Schapira AH. Progress in neuroprotection in Parkinson's disease. Eur J Neurol 2008;15(suppl 1):5–13.

20. Olanow CW, Hauser RA, Jankovic J, et al. A randomized, double-blind, placebo-controlled, delayed start study to assess rasagiline as a disease modifying therapy in Parkinson's disease (the ADAGIO study): rationale, design, and baseline characteristics. Mov Disord 2008; 23:2194–2201.

21. Hart RG, Pearce LA, Ravina BM, et al. Neuroprotection trials in Parkinson's disease: systematic review. Mov Disord 2009; 24:647–654.

22. Laitinen LV, Bergenheim AT, Hariz MI. Leksell's posteroventral pallidotomy in the treatment of Parkinson's disease. J Neurosurg 1992; 76:53–61.

23. Benabid AL , Chabardès S, Seigneuret E, et al. Surgical therapy for Parkinson's disease. J Neural Transm 2006; 70(suppl):383–392.

24. Limousin P, Martinez-Torres I. Deep brain stimulation for Parkinson's disease. Neurotherapeutics 2008;5:309–319.

25. Zeng X, Cai J, Chen J, et al. Dopaminergic differentiation of human embryonic stem cells. Stem Cells 2004; 22:925–940.

26. Roy NS, Cleren C, Singh SK, et al. Functional engraftment of human ES cell-derived dopaminergic neurons enriched by coculture with telomerase-immortalized midbrain astrocytes. Nat Med 2006; 12:1259–1268.

27. Hagell P, Piccini P, Björklund A, et al. Dyskinesias following neural transplantation in Parkinson's disease. Nat Neurosci 2002; 5:627–628.

28. Kordower JH, Freeman TB, Snow BJ, et al. Neuropathological evidence of graft survival and striatal reinnervation after the transplantation of fetal mesencephalic tissue in a patient with Parkinson's disease. N Engl J Med 1995; 332:1118–1124.

29. Bakay RAE, Raiser CD, Subramaian T, et al. Implantation of Spheramine® in advanced Parkinson's disease. Front Biosci 2004; 9:592–602.

30. Reynolds H, Wilson-Barnett J, Richardson G. Evaluation of the role of the Parkinson's disease nurse specialist, Int J Nurs Stud 2000;37:337–349.

31. Findley LJ. The economic impact of Parkinson's disease. Parkinsonism Relat Disord 2007; 13(suppl):S8–12.

32. Hely MA, Reid GJW, Adena MA, et al. Sydney Multicenter Study of Parkinson's disease: The inevitability of dementia at 20 years. Mov Disord 2008; 23:837–844.

33. Hoehn M, Yahr M. Parkinsonism: onset, progression and mortality. Neurology 1967; 17:427–442.
34. Sugawara A, Ohta M, Maeda T, et al. Mutual relationship between prevalence statistics and mortality statistics in Parkinson's disease. Nippon Eiseigaku Zasshi 2007; 62:64–69.
35. Hely MA, Morris JG, Reid WG, Trafficante R. Sydney Multicenter Study of Parkinson's disease: non-L-dopa-responsive problems dominate at 15 years. Mov Disord 2005; 20:1255–1263.
36. Hely MA, Reid WG, Adena MA, et al. The Sydney multicenter study of Parkinson's disease: the inevitability of dementia at 20 years. Mov Disord. 2008; 23:837–844.
37. Diem-Zangerl A, Seppi K, Wenning GK, et al. Mortality in Parkinson's disease: a 20 yr follow up study. Mov Disord 2009; 24:819–825.
38. Korell M, Tanner C. Epidemiology of Parkinson's disease:an overview. In: Ebadi M, Pfeiffer R, eds. Parkinson's Disease. Florida: CRC Press, 2005: 39–50.
39. Mylne A, Griffiths C, Rooney C, Doyle P. Trends in Parkinson's disease related mortality in England and Wales, 1993–2006. Eur J Neurol 2009; in press.

Chapter 2

Parkinsonian syndromes

K Ray Chaudhuri and Prashanth Reddy

Introduction

A variety of conditions may cause parkinsonian syndromes independent of the idiopathic loss of substantia nigra neurons and deafferentation of the striatum; these include degenerative conditions, infections, drugs, toxins and structural lesions (Figure 2.1). The clinical pictures of these degenerative conditions overlap but are usually recognized by the presence of subtle "red flags" in the earlier stage of the illness. Over the period of a few years a distinctive atypical clinical picture, separate to that of Parkinson's disease, emerges and is typically characterized by a poorer response to dopaminergic therapy. However, it may be impossible to distinguish idiopathic Parkinson's disease from other parkinsonian syndromes by clinical features alone, although review of the patient's medical history and diagnostic tests, such as sophisticated neuroimaging, can aid diagnosis [1].

Neurodegeneration-linked parkinsonism

Clinically, the most relevant conditions are multiple system atrophy (MSA), progressive supranuclear palsy (PSP), dementia with Lewy bodies (DLB) and corticobasal degeneration (CBD). There are rarer neurodegeneration-linked forms of parkinsonism such as those linked to Machado–Joseph disease (spinocerebellar ataxia [SCA] type 3), parkinsonism linked to Huntington's disease and neuronal brain iron accumulation syndromes (see Figure 2.1). Common and clinically relevant nondegenerative parkinsonian syndromes include vascular pseudoparkinsonism and drug-induced parkinsonism (DIP) and are discussed in this chapter.

Although the initial presenting symptoms may mimic Parkinson's disease with the presence of bradykinesia, occasional tremor and gait difficulties, the following symptoms favor a parkinsonian syndrome, also referred to as Parkinson-plus syndromes:

1. Lack of a meaningful response to oral levodopa or dopamine agonists in the early stages of the disease.

2. Early onset of postural instability leading to falls, autonomic symptoms such as postural hypotension, erectile failure and incontinence, usually within 2 years of onset of illness.

3. Presence of ocular signs, such as blinking on saccadic eye movements, a slow latency to downgaze, supranuclear gaze palsy (SNGP), square-wave jerks, nystagmus, blepharospasm and apraxia of eyelid opening or closure.

4. Presence of symmetrical signs in early stages of the disease with a dominance of truncal symptoms.

5. Early onset (usually within 1 year of onset of illness) of visual hallucinations or psychosis, either in the drug-naïve state or precipitated by low doses of levodopa or dopamine agonists.

Causes of parkinsonian syndromes

Degenerative parkinsonian syndromes
Multiple system atrophy (MSA-C, MSA-P)
Progressive supranuclear palsy (PSP-P,
  Richardson's syndrome, pure akinesia
  with gait freezing)
Dementia with Lewy bodies (DLB)
Corticobasal degeneration (CBD)
Parkinsonism linked to Alzheimer's disease
Hereditary degenerative diseases
Autosomal dominant cerebellar ataxias
  (Machado–Joseph disease SCA-3)
Neuronal brain iron accumulation syndromes
  (types 1 and 2, neuroferritinopathy, L-ferritin
  and PANK2 mutations, aceruloplasminemia)
Prion disorders
Hereditary frontotemporal dementias
Huntington's disease (juvenile Westphal variant,
  late-onset minimal chorea)
Neuroacanthocytosis
Wilson's disease
Whipple's disease
X-linked dystonia–parkinsonism (Lubag)
Parkinsonism–dementia–amyotrophic lateral
  sclerosis complex (Guam)
Atypical unclassifiable parkinsonism in Guadeloupe
Atypical presentation of genetic forms of
  parkinsonism:
  Kufor–Rakeb disease
  Glucocerebroxidase mutation-linked parkinsonism

Infections
Prion disease
HIV-related parkinsonism
Encephalitis lethargica

Toxins
MPTP, carbon monoxide, carbon
  disulfide, manganese, paraquat,
  hexane, rotenone and toluene

**Structural lesions
(mostly isolated case reports)**
Hydrocephalus
Falx cerebrii/motor strip
  meningioma
Cavernoma
Arteriovenous malformation
Infective cysts/tumors of
  basal ganglia (toxoplasmosis,
  cysticercosis)

Cerebrovascular disorders
Vascular pseudoparkinsonism

Figure 2.1 Causes of parkinsonian syndromes. MPTP, 1-methyl-4-phenyl-1,2,3,6-tetrahydropyridine; SCA, spinocerebellar ataxia.

Multiple system atrophy

MSA is a condition often confused with Parkinson's disease and usually presents with a variable combination of akinesia-dominant parkinsonism with autonomic, pyramidal or cerebellar symptoms and signs [2]. The prevalence is about 2–7/100,000 person-years. Historically, this condition was recognized as striatonigral degeneration (SND) when there were dominant parkinsonian signs, as olivopontocerebellar (OPCA) type if cerebellar signs predominated and as Shy–Drager syndrome if autonomic signs such as postural hypotension were dominant.

Quinn in 1989 and 1994, and subsequently Gilman et al. in 1998 and, most recently in 2008, the NNIPPS (Neuroprotection and Natural History in Parkinson Plus Syndromes) study group have formulated and refined criteria for diagnosis of MSA - the variant previously known as SND is now known as MSA-P, while the OPCA variant is called MSA-C and the term Shy–Drager syndrome is no longer in use [2–4]. The pathological feature of MSA is the glial cytoplasmic inclusions (argylophilic inclusions in the cytoplasm of oligodendroglia), although clinically the MSA-P phenotype presents the most difficulty in differentiating it from Parkinson's disease. Diagnostic categories include possible, probable and definite MSA (Figure 2.2). The parkinsonian features of MSA include progressive bradykinesia, which is usually symmetrical, rigidity and postural instability that leads to early and often en bloc falls; "red flags" that would raise the suspicion of MSA include disproportionate, and dystonic, anterocollis, truncal dystonias such as the Pisa syndrome, characteristic sighing, inspiratory stridors particularly at night, mini-myoclonus of fingers masquerading as tremor and the presence of cold, blue hands [4]. Autonomic failure in the form of sympathetic dysfunction occurs early in MSA, is more severe than in idiopathic Parkinson's disease and is often manifest as progressive postural hypotension, while genitourinary problems such as erectile failure may be prominent. Urinary symptoms may be very common and some argue that the urogenital form of MSA should have a separate subclassification since neurogenic dysfunction of the lower urinary tract may precede the diagnosis.

The diagnostic categories of multiple system atrophy (MSA)		
Possible MSA	**Probable MSA**	**Definite MSA**
Autonomic/urinary dysfunction or parkinsonism or cerebellar dysfunction + two features from other domains	Autonomic/urinary dysfunction + parkinsonism with poor levodopa response or cerebellar dysfunction	Pathologically confirmed MSA

Figure 2.2 The diagnostic categories of multiple system atrophy (MSA).

Urinary retention is common and urodynamic testing reveals a combination of detrusor hyperreflexia and urethral sphincter weakness. Magnetic resonance imaging (MRI) of the brain may reveal hypointensity, lateral margination of the putamen or an abnormal cross sign – the "hot cross bun" sign in the pons caused by the prominence of the transverse pontine fibers and atrophy of the pons (Figures 2.3 and 2.4). SPECT (single photon emission computed tomography) of the heart using the ligand MIBG (^{131}I-labeled *meta*-iodobenzylguanidine) may show early visualization of the heart in MSA (Figure 2.5), indicating intact peripheral sympathetic innervations of the heart; this is in contrast to what is usually observed in Parkinson's disease, where these innervations are usually impaired leading to nonvisualization of the heart. The use of neurophysiological techniques such as external anal and urethral sphincter electromyography (SEMG) remains controversial. This test is based on anterior horn cell loss in the nucleus of Onufrowicz in the sacral spinal cord in MSA. MSA does not usually have a genetic cause, although there have been reports of autosomal -dominant patterns in families.

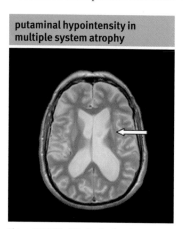

putaminal hypointensity in multiple system atrophy

Figure 2.3 MRI of the brain showing putaminal hypointensity in multiple system atrophy.

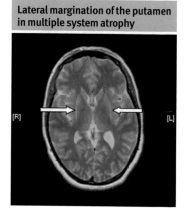

Lateral margination of the putamen in multiple system atrophy

Figure 2.4 MRI of the brain showing lateral margination of the putamen in multiple system atrophy.

Clinical signs/symptoms that would contradict a diagnosis of MSA include:

- Onset before 30 years of age
- Strong family history
- Early hallucinations unrelated to medication
- Early dementia
- Early vertical SNGP
- Cortical dysfunction such as aphasia and apraxia.

Uptake of MIBG showing intact peripheral sympathetic nervous system innervation of the heart in multiple system atrophy

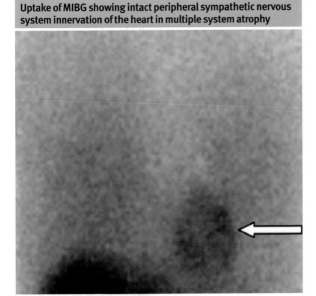

Figure 2.5 MIBG scan showing uptake of MIBG by the intact peripheral sympathetic nervous system innervation of the heart in MSA.

In MSA, there is a variable response to levodopa, and in MSA-P the benefit usually declines within 1–2 years of treatment [2,5]. High doses of levodopa may be required (up to 1.5–2 g/day). Often patients develop dyskinesia involving only the face and head. Treatment is otherwise symptomatic and centers on concentrated multidisciplinary care. The NNIPPS study reported the drug riluzole has no disease-modifying effect [4]. The lifespan is shorter compared with Parkinson's disease and patients may survive 6–8 years after diagnosis.

Progressive supranuclear palsy

PSP is also known as the Steele–Richardson–Olszewski syndrome and is a relentlessly progressive illness that usually presents with gait disturbance and leads to falls (backwards or sideways) in over 50% of cases within 1–2 years of diagnosis; it is a disease of later life starting in the late 50s or 60s [6]. The prevalence is similar to MSA and, in Europe, PSP is thought to make up 2–6% of parkinsonian patients seen in the clinic. High prevalence is noted in the French Antilles. However, unlike MSA and Parkinson's disease, which are synucleinopathies, the pathological hallmark of PSP is the presence of tau protein-positive filamentous inclusions, known as neurofibrillary tangles, in the glia and neurons.

In typical cases of PSP, the clinical picture consists of SNGP, particularly downgaze with severe neck rigidity causing the neck to be fixed in extension, often with a fixed "staring" look (reptilian stare); the "applause sign" (clapping in excess of three times when asked to copy three hand claps); and a predominant truncal extensor rigidity. Varying degrees of dysarthria, bradykinesia, dysphagia, personality changes and other behavioral disturbances, such as a subcortical frontal dementia and emotional lability, may coexist. "Rocket sign", where the patient jumps instinctively from a sitting position and falls back on the chair, occurs because of a combination of subcorticofrontal dysfunction and postural instability. Eye-movement abnormalities (external ocular movements) are common and often (but not always) present at the onset of the illness, and patients rarely die without developing SGNPs. The external ocular movements consist of square-wave jerks, instability of fixation, slow or hypometric saccades and, predominantly, SNGP, which clinically leads to a characteristic inability to look up or down to command. However, the restricted movements can be overcome by the doll's head reflex, where the eye moves to compensate for movements of the head, which is retained until very late. In the limbs, resting tremor is rare but has been reported, although the presence of unilateral resting tremor would favor a diagnosis of Parkinson's disease.

Several clinical variants of PSP have been described [6,7]. These include the classic Richardson's syndrome phenotype, which is associated with SNGP, nuchal rigidity and early falls; a parkinsonian variant of PSP, PSP-P, which is characterized by a variable response to levodopa, longer survival and lower tau pathology load in the brain; and the pure akinesia with gait freezing phenotype, in which patients do not show cognitive impairment or falls within the first 2 years of diagnosis. Cognitive problems dominate Richardson's phenotype and include progressive dementia that resembles Alzheimer's disease and can be confused with other tauopathies such as frontotemporal dementia, corticobasal degeneration or Pick's disease. The clinical heterogeneity of PSP is shown in Figure 2.6.

Atypical "variants" of progressive supranuclear palsy (PSP) or conditions in which PSP phenotype has been reported

Pure akinesia	Frontotemporal dementia and
Pure akinesia with gait freezing	motor neuron disease
Parkinsonian variant of PSP (PSP-P)	Creutzfeldt–Jakob disease
Severe dementia	Primary antiphospholipid
Unilateral limb dystonia and apraxia	antibody syndrome
Palatal tremor and cricopharyngeal dysfunction	Clebopride exposure
Frontotemporal dementia linked to chromosome 17	Whipple's disease

Figure 2.6 Atypical "variants" of progressive supranuclear palsy (PSP) or conditions in which PSP phenotype has been reported. Cerebral autosomal dominant anteriopathy with subcortical infarcts and leukoencephalopathy. (CADASIL)

Seven diagnostic criteria for PSP have been published, with those of the National Institute of Neurological Disorders and the Society for Progressive Supranuclear Palsy (NINDS–SPSP) being the most rigorous [6]. Diagnosis remains largely clinical, with diagnostic criteria having been recently refined by the NNIPPS study group. A number of families with clinically heterogeneous forms of PSP have been described. In the brain of someone with PSP, there appears to be a preponderance of four repeat tau gene isoforms, whereas a normal brain shows a dominance of three repeats. Mutation in the tau gene (MAPT) has been described. MRI of the brain can attempt to distinguish PSP from Parkinson's disease, in that the midbrain tectum and tegmentum atrophy in advanced supranuclear palsy and the "humming bird sign" may be observed [1]. Patients die within 5–10 years as a result of increasing bulbar problems and immobility.

Dementia with Lewy bodies

DLB presents with early onset dementia (progressive cognitive decline and behavioral abnormalities that may interfere with normal social and occupational function), and visual hallucinations, delusions and even psychosis in the drug-naïve state or usually within 1–2 years of diagnosis [8]. The condition may be indistinguishable in the early stages from Parkinson's disease and pathologically there is widespread deposition of Lewy bodies in the neocortex as well as in the brain-stem and diencephalic neurons. In some patients neurofibrillary tangles may be seen and indicate coincidental Alzheimer's disease. Of all cases of dementia reaching autopsy, 20% may have DLB. Autopsy findings in cases of DLB are inseparable from those in cases of dementia occurring late in Parkinson's disease (Parkinson's disease dementia).

Based on the opinion on an expert consensus group, clinical criteria for diagnosis were developed in 1996 and subsequently updated [9]. The revised criteria for diagnosis of DLB include a central feature, core features, suggestive features, supportive features and temporal sequence of symptoms (Figure 2.7). The characteristic "core features" of DLB include fluctuations in cognition and attention, recurrent and persistent visual hallucinations, and parkinsonian motor signs of bradykinesia, tremor and gait difficulties. Similar to PSP, falls may occur early and some patients are very sensitive to small doses of neuroleptics. Rarely, patients develop SNGP, which may lead to the condition being mistaken for PSP, while the pattern of early dementia may cause patients to be diagnosed with Alzheimer's disease.

Levodopa response is present in DLB but typically tails off with time unlike in Parkinson's disease, and the response to dopamine agonists is erratic, often being associated with early neuropsychiatric side effects. The electroencephalography (EEG) recording in DLB may be abnormal with background posterior slowing and frontally dominant burst activity, which is not a feature of Parkinson's disease. A DaT Scan may be useful in distinguishing DLB from Alzheimer's disease (Figure 2.8), in which the presynaptic DaT Scan is normal.

Revised criteria for diagnosis of dementia with Lewy bodies (DLB)

Central feature	Dementia
Core features	Fluctuating cognition Recurrent visual hallucinations Parkinsonism
Suggestive features	Rapid eye movement sleep behavior disorder Neuroleptic sensitivity Reduced striatal dopamine transporter activity on DaT scan

Supportive features	Repeated falls/syncope
	Severe dysautonomia
	Nonvisual hallucinations
	Transient loss of consciousness
	Delusions, depression
	Imaging abnormalities:
	    Medial temporal lobe structure preservation (MRI/CT scan)
	    Low MIBG cardiac uptake
	    Low uptake on SPECT/PET perfusion scans
	Prominent slow-wave EEG with temporal sharp waves

Unlikely features of DLB	Features of active cerebrovascular disease, appearance of parkinsonism after severe dementia Concurrent severe physical illness
Temporal sequence of symptoms	Dementia occurring before or together with parkinsonism

Figure 2.7 Revised criteria for diagnosis of dementia with Lewy bodies (DLB). CT, computed tomography; EEG, electroencephalography; MIBG, ^{131}I-labeled *meta*-iodobenzylguanidine; MRI, magnetic resonance imaging; PET, positron emission tomography; SPECT, single photon emission computed tomography.

DaT scan showing bilaterally reduced uptake in the striatum in dementia with Lewy bodies

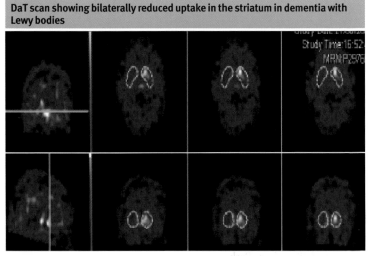

Figure 2.8 DaT scan showing bilaterally reduced uptake in the striatum in dementia with Lewy bodies (DLB). Courtesy of Dr M Buxton-Thomas.

Corticobasal degeneration

CBD is also known as corticobasal ganglionic degeneration or corticodentatonigral degeneration with neuronal achromasia. This is a rare condition (estimated incidence of 0.02–0.92/100,000 population per year) which typically presents in the sixth or seventh decade with slowly progressive, unilateral development of tremor, apraxia and rigidity in an upper limb (Figure 2.9). Patients then develop progressive gait disturbances, cortical sensory loss, motor apraxia and stimulus-sensitive myoclonus, which results in a jerky, uncontrollable hand. In 50% of patients, a jerky, uncontrollable movement of the lower extremity may develop and is known as the alien limb phenomenon. Mirror movements may occur and a slightly wide-based, apraxic gait is observed, similar to normal pressure hydrocephalus rather than the typical festinating gait of Parkinson's disease. After several years, the condition becomes bilateral with progressive cognitive impairment. Levodopa or other forms of dopaminergic treatment are ineffective and the disease course is relentlessly progressive.

The condition is associated with tau deposition in the brain and tau-containing filamentous inclusions in basal and cortical neurons. There are also swollen cortical neurons – "achromatic neurons". Phenotypic variability has been described and variants include early onset dementia and aphasia, frontotemporal dementia, and visuospatial and visuoperceptive deficits. MRI of the brain may show focal atrophy, particularly in the parietal areas, and positron emission tomography (PET) shows an asymmetric decrease in regional cerebral glucose metabolic rates.

Vascular pseudoparkinsonism

Vascular disease of the brain may lead to a parkinsonian syndrome, usually referred to as vascular pseudoparkinsonism (VP), that has a variety of clinical presentations. Onset of the illness may be acute or subacute and symptoms are usually bilateral, unlike in Parkinson's disease, and include rest tremor, bradykinesia, rigidity and postural instability. The disease course is dependent on the degree of vascular disease and may remain stable from onset of illness or progress gradually or, rarely, may resolve spontaneously. Most patients have predominant lower-extremity symptoms, such as a gait disturbance (freezing, gait initiation failure, turning difficulties), with minimal upper-extremity symptoms (previously known as lower-body parkinsonism), or walk with small steps (marche à petit pas), which is characteristic of vascular disease. This may cause difficulty in distinguishing the condition from the pure akinesia gait-freezing variant of PSP or from Parkinson's disease with the phenotype of postural instability and gait difficulty.

Clinical aspects of corticobasal degeneration	
Tremor (70–80% of patients)	6–8 Hz
	Kinetic and postural
	Jerky
Myoclonus (50%)	With jerky tremor
	Distal muscles
	Action, postural or stimulus sensitive
Dystonia (40-70%)	Asymmetric and mostly in arms
	Axial dystonia infrequent
	Pain with dystonia
	Contractures
	Associated chorea
Ocular signs	Increased latency of horizontal saccades
	Poor initiation of rapid saccades
	Visuospatial dysfunction
Cortical	Apraxia
	Ideomotor most frequent
	Cortical sensory loss
	Dysphasia
	Alien limb phenomenon
	Pyramidal signs
	Illusions, delusions, disinhibition
Urinary	Decreased bladder capacity
	Detrusor over-activity

Figure 2.9 Clinical aspects of corticobasal degeneration [10].

Often additional signs, such as spasticity or extensor plantar reflexes, may be present and indicate pyramidal tract involvement. VP may be separated from Parkinson's disease by the following:

- Normal cardiac uptake of MIBG using SPECT (reduced uptake in Parkinson's disease)
- Normal or near-normal olfaction in VP (abnormal in Parkinson's disease)
- Normal colonic transit time in VP (59 h) (slow in Parkinson's disease)
- Evidence of severe vascular white matter disease (Figure 2.10) on MRI of the brain which may cause reduced uptake on DaT Scan [1].

It has been proposed that chronic subcortical ischemia secondary to hypertensive vascular disease might be responsible for the disorder, resulting in disconnection between basal ganglia and the supplementary motor area. Three pathological variants are recognized:

1. **Brain-stem vascular lesions associated with parkinsonism:** may respond to levodopa therapy and usually unilateral in onset.

2. **Parkinsonism, associated with basal ganglia lesions:** unilateral/asymmetric parkinsonism often with acute/subacute onset; may respond to levodopa therapy.

3. **Parkinsonism related to cerebral white matter lesions:** often associated with short stepping gait with or without freezing.

Dopaminergic therapy can be attempted and some patients may respond to high doses of levodopa, as in those with brain-stem or nigral lesions, for a short period of time.

Vascular disease of the brain causing vascular pseudoparkinsonism

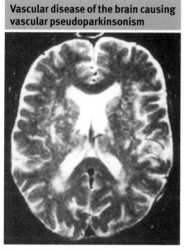

Figure 2.10 Vascular disease of the brain causing vascular pseudoparkinsonism. (Courtesy of Dr G MacPhee.)

Other parkinsonian syndromes

Postencephalitic parkinsonism

This is a disease that is believed to have been caused by a viral illness, stimulating degeneration of the nerve cells in the substantia nigra, and leading to clinical parkinsonism. The disease followed a condition called encephalitis lethargica (Von Economo's encephalitis) which was present during the influenza pandemic of 1918 – however, even using modern molecular diagnostic tests on human material from people who died at the time, no firm link between encephalitis lethargica and influenza has been made.

The brain regions affected contain neurofibrillary tangles, similar to those seen in Alzheimer's disease. However, the senile plaques observed in Alzheimer's disease are not found.

Dopa-responsive dystonia

Patients may develop young-onset parkinsonism with dominant dystonia, which may respond to dopaminergic drugs. Those with hereditary dopa-responsive dystonia caused by mutation in GTP cyclohydrolase (Segawa's disease) show a sustained and good response to low-dose levodopa. This disorder characteristically shows marked diurnal variation, with symptoms worsening as the day progresses, and may start in childhood with an odd and unusual gait, often with lower limb dystonia. PET and SPECT scans demonstrate markedly reduced 6-fluorodopa or DaT Scan uptake in patients with young-onset Parkinson's disease, while fluorodopa/DaT Scan uptake is normal in patients with dopa-responsive dystonia. Patients with dopa-responsive dystonia have a deficiency in the enzyme GTP cyclohydrolase, the genetic abnormality being on chromosome 14.

Lubag, an X-linked dystonia–parkinsonism found among Filipinos in the Capiz area in the island of Panay, also presents with dystonia and may develop into parkinsonism.

Wilson's disease

Wilson's disease should be considered in every case of young-onset parkinsonism, dystonia or indeed abnormal involuntary movements because this condition is treatable and the consequences of nonrecognition can be serious. The most common neurological manifestations include:

- asymmetric flapping arm tremor varying in amplitude and direction
- dystonia of face, arm and trunks
- rigidity
- cerebellar dysfunction with cerebellar gait and dysarthria (risus sardonicus is dystonia of the lower facial muscles)
- drooling of saliva
- ataxia.

Classically, the tremor is coarse, irregular and action-induced, and holding the arms forward and flexed horizontally may demonstrate the activity of the proximal muscles (wing-beating tremor).

Kayser–Fleischer rings – rings of brownish-green pigmentation due to copper deposition in the cornea – are best seen with a careful slit-lamp examination performed by an ophthalmologist. The condition is caused by a mutation in the

ATP7B gene, which results in an inability to transport copper to ceruloplasmin, leading to copper accumulation in the brain, liver, cornea and other areas.

Almost all patients with neurological features have MRI abnormalities in the basal ganglia. There is a pattern of symmetrical, bilateral, concentric-laminar T2 hyperintensity in the putamen, and involvement of the pars compacta of the substantia nigra, periaqueductal gray matter, pontine tegmentum and thalamus.

The most useful diagnostic test results are a low serum ceruloplasmin level and a raised 24-hour urinary copper excretion. Slit-lamp examination should be performed looking for Kayser–Fleischer rings (see above). Not all patients have a low ceruloplasmin level because inflammation, infection or oral contraceptive use may cause false elevations. Liver biopsy to show copper deposition remains the gold-standard diagnostic test.

Juvenile Huntington's disease

Juvenile Huntington's disease is an autosomal dominant neurodegenerative disorder known as the Westphal variant of the disease, which affects young people and may resemble parkinsonism. Onset is younger than 20 years and eye movement abnormalities, including apraxia, distinguish juvenile Huntington's disease from Parkinson's disease. Gene testing for Huntington's disease (which may show a cytosine, adenine and guanine [CAG] expansion of more than 35 trinucleotides) should be performed in all patients with juvenile-onset Parkinson's disease, and in adults with unusual features and cognitive decline. Late-onset parkinsonian Huntington's disease with levodopa responsiveness has also been described. Parkinsonism may also complicate the Huntington's disease-like syndrome type 2 (HDL2), which is associated with a mutation in the junctophilin-3 gene on chromosome 16.

Other parkinsonian syndromes associated with dystonia are listed in Figure 2.11.

Management

The management of the conditions listed in this chapter remains supportive. In neurodegeneration-linked parkinsonism, such as MSA-P, PSP-P and DLB, a trial of levodopa is often warranted and useful for a while at the maximum tolerated dose. Dopa-responsive dystonia responds to even small doses of levodopa. Cognitive impairments and psychosis need to be appropriately addressed and patients with DLB in particular may be very sensitive to neuroleptic effects. Cholinesterase inhibitors are useful in DLB but anticholinergics are best avoided. Myoclonus may be helped by clonazepam, whereas baclofen and tizanidine are useful for rigidity. Rapid eye movement behavior disorder may complicate MSA and DLB, and responds to clonazepam or melatonin. Zolpidem, a GABA-ergic drug (where GABA is γ-aminobutyric acid), has been reported to improve motor function and saccadic eye movements in PSP. The NNIPPS study group [4] reported that riluzole, an anti-glutamate agent, showed no disease-modifying effect in PSP or MSA. Multidisciplinary therapy is crucial for help with swallowing, posture, balance, fall prevention and limb function. Botulinum toxin therapy may be useful for contractures related to rigidity and drooling of saliva, and anticholinergics may help dystonia.

Parkinsonism associated with dystonic posturing and dystonia

Degenerative
Postencephalitic parkinsonism (often associated with dementia)
PSP
CBD
MSA
Frontotemporal dementia and parkinsonism (chromosome 17 linked)
Neuronal intermediate filament disease (dementia with corticospinal features)

Dystonic syndromes
Lubag (DYT3)
Dopa-responsive dystonia (DYT5, DYT14)
Rapid-onset dystonia parkinsonism (DYT12)

Inherited mixed pattern movement disorders
Juvenile Huntington's disease (also late-onset parkinsonian Huntington's disease with minimal chorea)
Huntington's disease-like syndrome type 2
Spinocerebellar ataxia and dentatorubro-pallidoluysian atrophy
SCA-3 (Machado–Joseph disease)
SCA-17
SCA-2 (only levodopa-responsive parkinsonism reported)
Neuroferritinopathy
Fahr's disease (idiopathic basal ganglia calcification)
McLeod's syndrome (X-linked neuroacanthocytosis syndrome)
Chorea acanthocytosis
Wilson's disease
Aceruloplasminemia
Pantothenate kinase-associated neurodegeneration (PANK-2 mutation on chromosome 20)
Gangliosidosis (GM1, GM2)
Niemann–Pick disease type C
Gaucher's disease type III (glucocerebrosidase gene mutations)
Glutaric aciduria
Homocystinuria
Neuronal ceroid lipofuscinoses
Biotin-responsive basal ganglia disease
Intranuclear hyaline inclusion disease

Sporadic disease
Drug-induced parkinsonism
Alzheimer's disease

Figure 2.11 Parkinsonism associated with dystonic posturing and dystonia. CBD, corticobasal degeneration; MSA, multiple system atrophy; PSP, progressive supranuclear palsy; SCA, spinocerebellar ataxia.

Conclusions

A wide range of conditions – degenerative, drug induced, vascular and metabolic – may cause a Parkinsonian syndrome that may mimic Parkinson's disease clinically. Occasionally, it may be impossible to distinguish between these conditions in life; however, advances in our understanding of the natural history and imaging techniques have improved the correct diagnosis rate, with important implications for prognosis and therapy. However, therapeutic options for many of these conditions – such as multiple system atrophy, Dementia with Lewy bodies and progressive supranuclear palsy – remain key unmet needs in the field of movement disorders.

References

1. Chaudhuri KR. Can we establish a definitive diagnosis of Parkinson's disease in life? In: Findley L, Hurwitz B, Miles A (eds), The Effective Management of Parkinson's Disease. London: Aesculapius Medical Press, 2004: 3–24.

2. Quinn NP. How to diagnose multiple system atrophy. Mov Disord 2005;20(suppl 12):S5–10.

3. Gilman S, Low PA, Quinn N, et al. Consensus statement on the diagnosis of multiple system atrophy. J Neurol Sci 1999;163:94–98.

4. Bensimon G, Ludolph A, Agid Y et al. Riluzole treatment, survival and diagnostic criteria in Parkinson plus disorders: The NNIPPS study. Brain 2009; 132:156–171.

5. Pfeiffer R. Multiple system atrophy. In: Aminoff MJ, Boller F, Swaab DF (series eds), Handbook of Clinical Neurology. Vol 84, Koller WC, Melamed E (eds), Parkinson's Disease and Related Disorders, Part II. Edinburgh: Elsevier, 2007: 307–26.

6. Burn DJ, Lees AJ. Progressive supranuclear palsy. In: Aminoff MJ, Boller F, Swaab DF (series eds), Handbook of Clinical Neurology. Vol 84, Koller WC, Melamed E (eds), Parkinson's Disease and Related Disorders, Part II. Edinburgh: Elsevier, 2007: 327–50.

7. Williams DR, Paviour DC, Watt HC, et al. Characteristics of two distinct clinical phenotypes observed in pathologically proven progressive supranuclear palsy: Richardson's syndrome and PSP-parkinsonism. Mov Disord 2004; 19:S328–329.

8. McKeith I. Dementia with Lewy bodies. In: Aminoff MJ, Boller F, Swaab DF (series eds), Handbook of Clinical Neurology. Vol 84, Koller WC, Melamed E (eds), Parkinson's Disease and Related Disorders, Part II. Edinburgh: Elsevier, 2007: 531–548.

9. McKeith I, Dickson D, Emre M, et al. Dementia with Lewy bodies: diagnosis and management: Third report of the DLB consortium. Neurology 2005; 65:1863–1672.

10. Stover NP, Walker HC, Watts RL. Corticobasal degeneration. In: Aminoff MJ, Boller F, Swaab DF (series eds), Handbook of Clinical Neurology. Vol 84, Koller WC, Melamed E (eds), Parkinson's Disease and Related Disorders, Part II. Edinburgh: Elsevier, 2007: 351–72.

Chapter 3

Dystonia

Rosalie Sherman and K Ray Chaudhuri

Definition

Dystonia refers to a group of neurological disorders characterized by spasmodic, patterned, repetitive or sustained co-contractions of agonist and antagonist muscle groups that eventually lead to abnormal twisting movements and postures. The movements range from slow twisting athetoid to rapid myoclonic jerky movements, and may occasionally be accompanied by a tremor [1]. The dystonic movements may be worse with movement (action dystonia), which is either nonspecific or task specific (eg, writer's cramp) [1].

Although genetic mutations and secondary causes, such as Wilson's disease, have been identified, most dystonic patients have idiopathic dystonia that has an unknown etiology [2,3]. The annual prevalence of idiopathic dystonia in Europe has been reported to be 15.2/100,000.

Classification

The etiologies and clinical manifestations of the dystonic syndromes are heterogeneous and encompass a large number of diseases [4]. Over the years, they have been classified according to a number of different categories including age of onset, site of affected area and, more recently, their genetic basis [2,5,6]. However, the most commonly used classifications are based on either the location of the dystonia or its pathophysiology.

Location

- **Focal dystonia** describes a dystonia where a single region of the body is involved:
  - writer's cramp: arm/forearm
  - blepharospasm: eyes
  - hemifacial spasm: face
  - cervical dystonia (also known as torticollis): neck
  - spasmodic dysphonia: larynx

– Meigs' syndrome: a mixture of above
- **segmental dystonia** describes a dystonia that includes two or more contiguous areas
    – craniocervical dystonia
    – crural dystonia: one leg and trunk/both legs
    – brachial dystonia: one arm and trunk/both arms.
- **Multifocal dystonia** includes all those disorders where more than two areas are affected; these are often in unrelated regions of the body.
- **Hemidystonia** refers to dystonia that is confined to only one side of the body. This usually follows a disease process such as a stroke.
- **Generalized dystonias** are much more severe and can affect the entire body. This is also referred to as primary torsion dystonia.

These are the most common forms of dystonia affecting 11.7/100,000 people annually in Europe [7]. Usually sporadic, they tend to appear in adult life and remain focal in distribution [1]. The most common focal dystonias are described here.

Cervical dystonia (spasmodic torticollis)

Spasmodic torticollis is the most common type of focal dystonia that presents to physicians. It affects around 10,000 people in the UK, for example. Its average age of onset is in the fifth decade and it affects more women than men [7]. This condition is characterized by spasms of the neck causing the head to turn uncontrollably to assume abnormal postures (Figure 3.1). Twisting of the head around the horizontal axis (torticollis) as a result of overactive contralateral sternomastoid and ipsilateral splenius capitis is the most common movement, present in 80% of patients. The head can also tilt to one side (laterocollis), back (retrocollis) or forward (antecollis) but these are less common. Pain is present in 75% and is the result of spasms or compression of nerves. This condition develops gradually and deteriorates over 5 years. At this point symptoms either stabilize or progress to segmental dystonia, which occurs in around a third of cases [6]. Long-term complications include cervical spine degeneration leading to radicular or myelopathic symptoms. Many patients develop sensory tricks to alleviate their symptoms. These include touching the back of the head, cheek or temple [1].

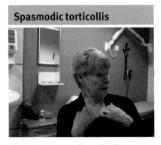

Spasmodic torticollis

Figure 3.1 Spasmodic torticollis.

Blepharospasm

Blepharospasm is the second most common dystonia, occurring in around 50,000 people in the USA, for example, with a larger proportion of these being women [7] (Figure 3.2). It is characterized by involuntary contraction of the orbicularis oris, which in its severe form prevents eyes from opening, rendering the patient functionally blind [1,7]. Onset is usually in the sixth or seventh decade and the dystonia develops insidiously, with the first signs being eye irritation and discomfort, light sensitivity and an increase in frequency of blinking. It often improves with talking or singing.

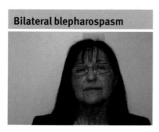

Bilateral blepharospasm

Figure 3.2 Bilateral blepharospasm.

Writer's cramp

Writer's cramp is the most common task-specific dystonia, with a prevalence of 69/100,000 in the USA, for example, and, in contrast to cervical dystonia, is more common in males than in females [7,8] (Figure 3.3). Onset is usually between the third and fifth decades and presents initially with tension and discomfort in the fingers and forearm that interferes with writing fluency. Patients find that they grip their pen too tightly and their writing becomes slow and untidy. Commonly this involves excessive flexion of the thumb and index finger with pronation of the hand and ulnar deviation of the wrist. This contraction disappears when the patient ceases writing. Up to 50% of patients also report either a tremor of the upper limb on writing or a postural tremor, but pain is an uncommon feature. Many patients develop strategies to overcome this cramp: they may support the hand with the opposite arm, use thick ribbed pens, alter grip or learn to write with nondominant hand. Unfortunately up to 10% of patients can develop cramp in this hand as well [9].

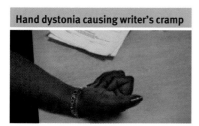

Hand dystonia causing writer's cramp

Figure 3.3 Hand dystonia causing writer's cramp.

Spasmodic dysphonia

Spasmodic dysphonia is relatively rare. It is more common in women and tends to appear in middle age. There are two types that are commonly seen [10]. The first is called the adductor type, which is the most common type. Speaking causes excessive involuntary spasms of thyroarytenoid and lateral cricoarytenoid muscles, bringing the vocal folds together. The voice quality is strained, strangled and choked, with a broken speech pattern, particularly with vowels, but the patient can often laugh, whisper and sing normally. The second is the abductor type, in which there is excessive contraction of posterior cricoarytenoid and cricothyroid muscles that separate the vocal folds. This produces a breathy, whispering voice pattern [1]. This dystonia may follow infections of the upper respiratory tract, injury to the larynx or excess voice use. Both types of spasmodic dystonia are speech-specific and a voice tremor may be present.

The condition may be seen in neurodegenerative disorders such as motor neuron disease, multiple system atrophy and Parkinson's disease.

Hemifacial spasm

Hemifacial dystonia affects around 4000 people in the UK with an onset in middle age. It appears to occur equally in both men and women but for unknown reasons presents predominantly on the left rather than the right side of the face (Figure 3.4).

It is characterized by the insidious onset of contraction of the facial muscles on just one side of the face. Initially the muscles around the eye are affected, and the contraction subsequently spreads to the jaw and mouth. Some patients have also reported a clicking sound in the ear with every muscle spasm. There is some speculation about whether or not this is a true dystonia, however, as it is also thought to be due to irritation of the facial nerve caused by an aberrant blood vessel.

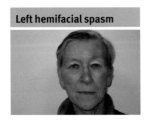

Left hemifacial spasm

Figure 3.4 Left hemifacial spasm.

Pathophysiology

The dystonia syndromes can also be classified according to the biological and physical manifestations of disease and are typically subdivided into primary torsion dystonia, secondary dystonia, heredodegenerative dystonia, dystonia plus and drug-induced dystonia [2,4,6]. These are shown in Figure 3.5.

Primary dystonia

Primary torsion dystonia (PTD) refers to those syndromes in which dystonia is the only symptom and there is no evidence of brain injury or any other possible cause. Many of these syndromes have a genetic basis [11]. Age and site of onset vary but are good prognostic factors for clinical progression.

Early onset PTD (onset around age 9) most commonly begins in the leg or arm and spreads to the other limb or trunk. This is also known as Oppenheim's dystonia or dystonia musculorum deformans and is linked to the *DYT1* gene on chromosome 9q34, which shows an autosomal dominant trait with a 30–40% reduced penetrance. In contrast late-onset PTD (onset around age 45 years) typically involves the upper body and most commonly remains focal or segmental [4].

Secondary dystonia

Secondary dystonia refers to conditions in which an identifiable cause for the dystonia is known [6]. Most of these conditions directly involve the basal ganglia and lead to a contralateral hemidystonia. Infarcts, tumors, vascular malformations and traumatic injuries to the basal ganglia are well-described causes but injury to cortical structures, the spinal cord and even peripheral nerves has also been linked with dystonia. Infectious, post-infectious and inflammatory syndromes associated with dystonia usually present with other movement disorders as well, such as parkinsonism, chorea, athetosis and tics [1].

The following are features that suggest that the dystonia is secondary:
- History of exogenous insult or exposure – drugs, head trauma, encephalitis
- Dystonia with rest (in PTD dystonia is worse with action)
- Atypical site for age of onset (leg onset in adult, cranial onset in child)
- Hemidystonia
- Continuous progression or symptoms
- Abnormalities on neurological examination: parkinsonism, ataxia, dementia, seizures, myoclonus, visual loss, dysarthria, Kayser–Fleisher rings, deafness, hepatosplenomegaly
- Abnormal brain scan or laboratory results
- Abnormal birth/perinatal history, developmental delay.

Heredodegenerative dystonia

Heredodegenerative dystonias are syndromes in which there is a neurodegenerative disease, with dystonia typically being a major feature. However, dystonia may not always be present. A large proportion of conditions in this subgroup have a genetic abnormality and they can be subdivided into disorders of metabolism, mitochondrial disease, trinucleotide repeat diseases, parkinsonian disorders and other degenerative processes [1].

Classification of dystonia syndromes by biological and physical disease manifestations

Type	Clinical picture	Examples
Primary dystonia	Dystonia (and perhaps tremor) is the only phenotypic manifestation with no identifiable cause	Early onset and late-onset types
Secondary dystonia	Inherited or acquired as a consequence of external factors, ie toxins or other diseases causing brain damage	**Cerebrovascular diseases** Stroke, hypoxia, CNS trauma, congenital malformations, intracranial hemorrhage **Infections** CJD, viral encephalitis **Other causes** SLE, Sjögren's syndrome, antiphospholipid syndrome, demyelinating or neoplastic, metabolic (hypoparathyroidism), cerebral palsy
Heredodegenerative	Neurodegenerative diseases with dystonia commonly being the major feature Many have a proven or possible genetic basis	**Metabolic disorders** *Metal-related disorders* Wilson's disease, neurodegeneration with brain iron accumulation (NBIA, type 1), neuroferritinopathy, Fahr's disease *Lysosomal storage disorders* Niemann–Pick disease type 3, Krabbe's disease, metachromatic leukodystrophy, GM1, GM2 gangliosidosis, Pelizaeus–Merzbacher disease *Acidurias* Glutaric aciduria type 1, Hartnup's disease, methylmalonic aciduria, propionic acidemia *Mitochondrial disorders* Leber's hereditary optic neuropathy, Leigh's disease, Mohr–Tranenberg syndrome **Trinucleotide repeat disorders** Huntington's disease, spinocerebellar ataxias, Huntington's disease-like syndromes **Parkinsonsim** Parkinson's disease Young-onset Parkinson's disease Progressive supranuclear palsy Multiple system atrophy Corticobasal degeneration Lubag Dementia with Lewy bodies
Dystonia plus	Syndromes with dystonia and neurological symptoms Neurochemical basis found but no evidence of degeneration	Alcohol-sensitive myoclic dystonia Dopa-responsive dystonia, rapid-onset dystonia–parkinsonism
Drug induced	Some may not actually cause the dystonia but may aggravate the pre-existing disorder	Antidepressants (SSRIs), neuroleptics, midazolam, phenytoin, verapamil, MAO inhibitors, flecainide, cocaine, ranitidine, levodopa, metoclopramide

Figure 3.5 Classification of dystonia syndromes by biological and physical disease manifestations. CJD, Creutzfeldt–Jakob disease; CNS, central nervous system; MAO, monoamine oxidase; SLE, systemic lupus erythematosus; SSRIs, selective serotonin reuptake inhibitors.

Dystonia-plus syndromes

The dystonia-plus subgroup was created to distinguish certain syndromes from the PTD and heredodegenerative dystonia subgroups [12]. These syndromes present with dystonia and other neurological symptoms but with no degenerative processes evident. The main conditions incorporated into this group are dystonia–parkinsonism syndrome, myoclonus–dystonia syndrome and dopa-responsive dystonia (DRD).

Dystonia–parkinsonism syndrome is a rare autosomal dominant movement disorder with reduced penetrance that develops in adolescence. It is characterized by acute onset (within days) of both dystonia and parkinsonism, with prominent bulbar involvement. Symptoms include dystonic posturing of limbs, bradykinesia, dysarthria and dysphagia. This can be preceded by stable mild limb dystonia for a number of years, and potential triggers are thought to be emotional trauma, extreme heat or physical exertion. Imaging of presynaptic dopamine uptake sites has been normal but some patients have shown reduced levels of cerebrospinal fluid (CSF) dopamine metabolites, and hence this disorder is believed to be a result of neuronal dysfunction rather than neuronal degeneration [1].

Myoclonus–dystonia syndrome refers to a condition where both myoclonus and dystonia coexist [13]. It usually starts in childhood or adolescence, with myoclonus affecting the upper limbs and axial muscles either at rest or in action. The dystonia appears to affect two-thirds of cases, presenting most commonly with writer's cramp or spasmodic torticollis. Relief is observed with both alcohol and benzodiazepines, often leading to abuse of these substances.

Dopamine-responsive dystonia is an inherited autosomal dominant trait with reduced penetrance. Patients most commonly present in childhood with gait problems related to foot dystonia, which worsens throughout the day and is relieved by rest [1,4]. Progression varies, with some patients developing generalized dystonia whereas others develop lower limb spasticity. Occasionally, dopamine-responsive dystonia may present with writer's cramp, spasmodic torticollis or parkinsonism features in adult life. The main characteristic of this syndrome is that there is a dramatic response to small doses of levodopa. Differential diagnoses include early onset primary torsion dystonia, spastic paraplegia and cerebral palsy, and early onset parkinsonism.

The myoclonus dystonia syndrome is characterized by dystonia (cervical dystonia, writer's cramps, leg dystonia) with almost 'lightning'-like myoclonic jerks aggravated by action, and is often inherited as a autosomal dominant triad with mutations in the ε-sarcoglycan (*DYT11*) gene. Another locus (*DYT15*) has been mapped to chromosome 18.

Rapid-onset dystonia parkinsonism (RDP) is a rare disorder in which there is abrupt or subacute onset of dystonia and parkinsonism over a period of hours to days. Bulbar involvement is common as is postural instability, dysarthria and marked bradykinesia but with little or no progression. Presymptomaptic dopamine neuronal imaging with PET is normal as is MRI of the brain. Emotional trauma, heat or physical exertion may precipitate the condition. The gene for this condition has been mapped to chromosome 19 (*DYT12*) and mutations in *ATP1A3* (Na$^+$/K$^+$ ATPase) have also been reported in seven unrelated kindreds.

Drug-induced dystonia

Drugs can cause transient or chronic (tardive) dystonia that appears to predominantly affect the face and neck. Acute dystonic reactions have been shown to follow treatment with dopamine-receptor-blocking drugs (neuroleptics, metoclopramide, prochlorperazine), antidepressants (selective serotonin reuptake inhibitors or monoamine oxidase inhibitors), calcium antagonists, general anesthetic agents, anticonvulsants (carbamazepine, phenytoin), levodopa, ranitidine, ecstasy and cocaine. In contrast, tardive dystonia, described as a dystonia lasting for at least 1 month, has been reported only after long-term use of dopamine-receptor-blocking drugs [1,4,12].

Epidemiology

The true prevalence of dystonia is relatively unknown. The prevalence figures available are usually based on studies of diagnosed cases only and therefore underestimate the real number because a significant number of cases of focal dystonia are undiagnosed or misdiagnosed [1]. A study by Defazio et al. [14] observed that the numbers of people with primary early onset and late-onset dystonia seeking medical attention, respectively, are 24–50 per million and 101–430 per million. Adjustment for possible underdiagnosis increases the estimates, for example to 600 per million for late-onset dystonia in the overall population of northern England. Results found in this study were reproduced in a number of other studies [15].

The most prevalent type of primary torsion dystonia is focal dystonia, of which cervical dystonia is the most common form with prevalence rates reported to be between 57 and 290 per million population. Rates for blepharospasm are 17–80 and 14–61 per million [1].

Genetics

It has long been thought that some of these sydromes may have a genetic element, because a large proportion of relatives of dystonia sufferers appear to acquire either tremors or dystonia-like symptoms. Following these findings studies have focused on possible genetic abnormalities that may lead to this phenomenon. To date around 13 dystonic syndromes have been differentiated by their genetic bases and their loci are known as *DYT1* to *DYT13* (Figure 3.6).

Dystonic syndromes and their loci			
Locus	**Chromosome**	**Type of dystonia**	**Inheritance**
DYT1	9	Early onset PTD	AD
DYT2	–	Autosomal recessive PTD	AR
DYT3 (Lubag)	X	X-linked dystonia–parkinsonism	AD
DYT4	–	'Non-DYT1' PTD	AD
DYT5/GCH1	14	Dopa-responsive dystonia	AD
DYT6	8	Adolescent-onset PTD	AD
DYT7	18	Adult-onset focal PTD	AD
DYT8	2	Paroxysmal dystonic choreoathetosis	AD
DYT9	1	Paroxysmal choreoathetosis with episodic ataxia and spasticity	AD
DYT10	16	Paroxysmal kinesiogenic choreoathetosis	AD
DYT11	7	Myoclonus–dystonia	AD
DYT12	19	Rapid-onset dystonia parkinsonism	AD
DYT13	1	Early and late-onset focal or segmental dystonia	AD

Figure 3.6 Dystonic syndromes and their loci. AD, autosomal dominant; AR, autosomal recessive; PTD, primary torsion dystonia. Modified from de Carvalho et al. [4].

DYT1

Currently, DYT1 dystonia is the most studied genetic dystonia. It was specifically studied in a population of Ashkenazi Jews where early onset dystonia seemed to occur more frequently, and it was mapped to chromosome 9q34 [4]. It is caused by a three base-pair deletion (GAG) in the *TORIA* gene, causing a loss of a glutamic acid residue in torsin A, the protein encoded by *DYT1*. This altered torsin A is thought to accumulate in the nuclear envelope of cells, causing membranous inclusions known as spheroid bodies in the cytoplasm. It is these spheroid bodies that appear to be associated with the pathogenesis of dystonia. In addition, both torsin A and its mRNA are highly expressed in dopaminergic neurons of the substantia nigra compacta, suggesting a dysfunction in dopamine transmission.

GCH1

Dopa-responsive dystonia (Segawa's disease) is an autosomal dominant condition caused by heterogeneous mutations in the *GCH1* gene located on chromosome 14 [16,17]. It varies in penetrance, with women acquiring the most penetrant version. GCH1 is the rate-limiting enzyme in the synthesis of tetrahydrobiopterin, which is a cofactor for phenylalanine, tryptophan and tyrosine (the rate-limiting enzyme in dopamine synthesis) [4]. The mutation causes a 20% decrease in GCH1 activity resulting in less dopamine being present in the nigrostriatal dopaminergic neurons. This is why dopamine-responsive dystonia improves so rapidly with levodopa treatment.

Lubag

X-linked dystonia–parkinsonism, also known as Lubag, was first described by Lee and colleagues [18] in the Philippines and mapped to chromosome Xq13. It is characterized by X-linked recessive inheritance with complete penetrance presenting by the fifth decade (mean onset is 37.9 years) [19]. It typically starts as a focal dystonia and becomes segmental in 22% and generalized in 78%. It may also develop parkinsonism symptoms in 50% of cases. Postmortem analyses of brain specimens have revealed neuronal loss and astrocytosis in the caudate nucleus and lateral putamen, which is why this syndrome is placed in the heredodegenerative subgroup, but the mechanism behind this is largely unknown and further studies are still in progress.

Signs and symptoms

Symptoms of dystonia result from the concurrent contractions of agonist and antagonist muscles that appear to follow a directional pattern but with varying speed and intensity. The majority of symptoms are very type-specific, (Figure 3.7) but there are a few common characteristics that apply to a large proportion of these syndromes:

- Abnormal posturing, especially on movement, that is improved with relaxation, sleep or 'sensory tricks' – touching the chin in cervical dystonia or touching the lateral canthus of the eye in blepharospasm
- Continuous pain
- Cramping or relentless muscle spasms.

History and investigations

There is no definitive test for dystonia because the diagnosis is largely a clinical one. However, specific tests are often done to confirm the diagnosis, exclude other diseases and find the primary cause of a secondary dystonia (Figure 3.8) [1].

It is important to establish whether there is a history of birth injury, family history of other neurological disorders or exposure to dystonia-inducing drugs.

Hemidystonia is highly suggestive of a contralateral lesion of the basal ganglia and magnetic resonance imaging (MRI) would be the first-line investigation.

Signs and symptoms of dystonia

Torticollis (twisting of the neck)	Laterocollis Rotational torticollis Retrocollis Myclonic torticollis Antecollis
Pain in the neck	Neck spasms
Hemifacial spasm	Initially ocular muscle spasms and then spread to mouth and jaw Left side affected more than the right Clicking sound in the ear on muscle contraction
Writer's cramp	Contraction or extension of the hand and forearm muscles Tension and discomfort on writing Writing becomes slow and untidy
Blepharospasm	Uncontrollable blinking Facial distortions and grimacing on attempting to open eyes Worse when tired, when stressed or when reading Functional blindness
Spasmodic dysphonia	Adductor type: strained, strangled and choked voice quality Broken speech pattern Abductor type: breathy, whispering voice quality

Figure 3.7 Signs and symptoms of dystonia.

Investigations for dystonia

Dystonia phenotype	Investigation
Primary torsion dystonia Early onset (<26 years)	Copper studies, slit-lamp examination MRI of the brain *DYT1* gene analysis Trial of levodopa
Late onset (>26 years)	Copper studies, slit-lamp if under 50 years MRI of the brain MRI of the spine if dystonia fixed or painful EMG if painful axial muscle spasm
Secondary dystonia	MRI of the brain/spine Nerve conduction studies Copper studies, slit-lamp, liver biopsy Genetic tests for neurodegenerative disorders, eg Huntington's disease, SCA, HD-linked syndromes White cell enzymes α-Fetoprotein, immunoglobulins Lactate, pyruvate, mtDNA analysis, muscle biopsy Fresh whole blood film for acanthocytes Urine amino acids, organic acids, oligosaccharides Bone marrow biopsy Phenylalanine loading test, CSF proteins ERG, retinal examination

Figure 3.8 Investigations for dystonia. CSF, cerebrospinal fluid; EMG, electromyogram; ERG, electroretinogram; HD, Huntington's disease; MRI, magnetic resonance imaging; mtDNA, mitochondrial DNA; SCA, spinocerebellar ataxia.

If MRI is normal, it may then be appropriate to exclude Wilson's disease using a slit-lamp examination, serum ceruloplasmin and 24-hour urinary copper excretion, and occasionally a liver biopsy.

Subsequent investigations for metabolic or heredodegenerative disorders may then be needed.

Psychogenic dystonia

This condition is difficult to diagnose and may cause marked disability. As there is a lack of diagnostic tests, the condition needs to be diagnosed by a multispecialty team incorporating a psychiatrist. Diagnostic features includes inconsistent signs and evidence of underlying stress disorders or psychiatric problems. The prognosis is poor and diagnosis may be delayed. Cognitive–behavioral therapy may be useful.

Treatments

The first step in treatment of dystonia is ruling out any underlying cause. In secondary dystonias it may be possible to cure the dystonia if the underlying cause is treated adequately (eg, Wilson's disease).

Although a number of genetic mutations and secondary etiologies are known, most patients have idiopathic dystonia, so specific pathogenesis-targeted treatment is available only for a very limited number of symptomatic dystonias, such as levodopa in dopa-responsive dystonia. As a result current treatment is predominantly targeted at relieving symptoms, with the aim of improving muscle function and dexterity, alleviating pain, correcting posture and improving quality of life.

There are various options available for the treatment of dystonia, which include oral medications, injections into the dystonic muscle and surgery. The choice of treatment depends on the severity and site of the dystonia. Looking at the literature it is possible to see that specific dystonic syndromes respond more effectively to particular modes of treatment than others [3,20]. Treatment options are summarized in Figure 3.9.

Medication

There have been a variety of drugs recommended for use in treatment of dystonia. They all act by inhibiting various different neurotransmitters in the nervous system that are responsible for execution and control of movement. The efficacy of individual medications may depend on the individual and the specific pathology of the dsytonia; for example, dystonia-responsive dystonia is known to respond to levodopa but most dystonias have an unknown pathophysiology and as such may require a trial and error of drugs or combination therapy. Oral therapy should only be used with careful consideration of the risk:benefit ratio.

Treatments for specific dystonic syndromes

Segmental dystonias
Anticholinergics, eg trihexyphenidyl, orphenadine, benzatropine, procycline
Benzodiazepines, e.g. diazepam, clonazepam, lorazepam, alprazolam
Baclofen
Dopamine agonists/antagonists
Tetrabenazine
Deep brain stimulation

Focal dystonias
Blepharospasm
Botulinum toxin injection
Benzodiazepines/anticholinergics
Myomectomy (very rarely performed in severe cases)

Oromandibular dystonia/writer's cramp
Botulinum toxin injection
Baclofen/anticholinergics

Spasmodic dysphonia
Botulinium toxin injection

Cervical dystonia
Botulinum toxin injections
Anticholinergics
Benzodiazepines
Baclofen
Peripheral surgical denervation of nerves supplying dystonic muscles or myectomy
Deep brain stimulation of the internal segment of globus pallidus

Figure 3.9 Treatments for specific dystonic syndromes.

Anticholinergic agents

These drugs inhibit the action, release and production of the neurotransmitter acetylcholine, which is responsible for activating muscles. The effectiveness of these drugs, specifically trihexyphenidyl, has been documented in focal, segmental and generalized dystonias [21–24]. One prospective placebo-controlled trial found that 67% of patients with early onset primary dystonia improved and continued to benefit after 2.4 years [25]. However, it appears to be less useful in adults, which is thought to be because higher doses are less well tolerated and doses up to 100 mg/day may have to be used [2]. Greater benefit is also seen if therapy is started early on in the disease process, although this is seen in both children and adults [25]. There are issues with tolerability of these drugs because side effects such as dry mouth, blurred vision, constipation, memory impairment and confusion can be quite severe, especially at high doses. However, side effects can be minimized by increasing the dose in a stepwise manner.

Benzodiazepines

This class of drug regulates GABA (γ-aminobutyric acid), an excitatory transmitter that helps the brain maintain muscle control. It binds to specific benzodiazepine receptor and increases its affinity for GABA, causing postsynaptic neuron hyperpolarization. Benzodiazepines are specifically indicated for use in focal dystonias and in our opinion help around 20% of those with spasmodic torticollis. However, most studies have failed to document a dramatic or sustained benefit from use of these drugs and it has been suggested that it may be the mild sedation that accounts for the improvement in symptoms observed [1]. Nonetheless, they do still benefit the occasional patient quite dramatically [26] and so continue to be prescribed specifically as an adjunct to anticholinergics. The presence of side effects depends on the dose used but the most common effects are drowsiness, confusion and light-headedness.

Baclofen

This is a structural analog of GABA that reduces spinal cord interneuron and motor neuron excitability. A retrospective study found that it was especially beneficial and better tolerated in early onset primary dystonia [2] but had minimal effects in late-onset primary dystonia [1]. Significant side effects such as lethargy, dizziness and confusion have been documented.

Occasionally a combination of trihexyphenidyl, baclofen and benzodiazepines may be necessary.

Intrathecal baclofen pump

This device works by injecting a therapeutic dose of baclofen via a pump directly into the spinal fluid. Clinical efficacy is seen at much lower doses than are seen with oral administration, and sedation is minimized. Again, response is varied with some significant benefit seen in secondary generalized dystonia and in patients with dystonia and spasticity [27,28], but its efficacy seems to be limited to certain syndromes and in specific symptomatic dystonias its effect is fairly minimal.

It is preferred over oral baclofen in severe resistant dystonia or aggravated dystonia, but there may be problems with side effects, infection and equipment.

Dopaminergic agents (eg, levodopa, bromocriptine, amantadine)

The dopaminergic drug levodopa is frequently trialed in childhood/young-onset dystonias, as around 5% of these are dopa-responsive dystonias, that show a dramatic response to low doses of levodopa (with decarboxylase inhibitor)

[3,29]. As explained above, dopa-responsive dystonia is associated with a genetic mutation in the gene for GTP cyclohydrolase 1, which is required in the synthesis of dopamine, and levodopa crosses the blood–brain barrier and is metabolized to dopamine to negate the effects of dopamine deficiency. Many studies have suggested that variable doses ranging from 100 to 1000 mg daily may be efficacious [1,3].

Dopamine antagonists
(eg, phenothiazines, haloperidol, tetrabenazine, clozapine)
Paradoxically, dopamine antagonists and dopamine-depleting agents have also been used in the past but their use is now discouraged because of their side effects, notably parkinsonism and tardive dyskinesia.

Botulinum toxin injection
Botulinum toxin injection [20] has been used since the 1980s and is the first-line treatment for those patients with focal and segmental dystonia. Botulinum neurotoxin type A, which is the most commonly used, is one of seven different serotypes of botulinum toxin that act through inhibiting calcium ion-mediated release of acetylcholine at the motor nerve terminals. Acetylcholine is a neurotransmitter responsible for activation of muscle contraction, and so inhibiting its release results in the muscle being temporarily paralyzed. Double-blind, placebo-controlled trials have shown that these injections are efficacious in treating blepharospasm and cervical dystonia, resulting in a 60% improvement in symptoms [1,30]. In addition further trials have demonstrated their use for laryngeal dystonia, writer's cramp and limb dystonias. Botulinum toxin is diluted and injected into the muscles that are painful, tender and visibly contracting, and also into muscles that may contribute to the abnormal movement.

The effects of botulinum toxin are usually greatest for a 2- to 6-week period but as nerve endings grow back after 8 weeks the effects of the toxin wear off, requiring injections to be repeated every 2–3 months. There are no permanent side effects associated with this treatment, but immediately after the injection there may be localized discomfort or pain for a few days. There are also specific side effects of the injection at specific sites (eg, ptosis/double vision with eyelid injection, dysphagia with cervical muscle injection, soft speech or dysphagia in vocal fold injection).

Another problem is the development of resistance to the toxin after repeated treatment, which occurs in around 10% of patients. Development of less antigenic forms of type A toxin or the use of other strains (B or F) may overcome this problem but this has yet to be shown clinically [31].

Surgery

The surgical approach tends to be reserved for those syndromes in which there is no response to traditional medical treatment and there is continued severe disabling dystonia. This form of treatment is becoming more popular because of improvements in functional anatomy, surgical techniques and imaging [3].

Recordings taken from the brains of patients with dystonia have revealed abnormal discharge rates and patterns in the basal ganglia with overactivity of pathways in the globus pallidus. Ablative surgery (pallidotomy) and deep brain stimulation (DBS) of the globus pallidus have both resulted in improvements in the symptoms of dystonia, which is most likely to be due to disruption of the abnormal discharge pattern and reduction of the cortical disinhibition that is associated with dystonia [32].

In a class III multicenter trial, patients with generalized dystonia who received bilateral palladial DBS showed a 54% improvement on the Burke–Fahn–Marsden scale [33]. These results were also shown to occur in secondary dystonia, cervical dystonia and tardive dystonia but to a lesser extent. Due to the efficacy of this treatment it is often used as a second-line treatment in primary generalized dystonia.

DBS appears to be largely replacing pallidotomy because there are fewer risks or side effects and it is a reversible procedure that can be more easily tailored to individual needs. However, problems with DBS include hardware and battery failure, high costs and the necessity for time-consuming follow up [1].

Other surgical options

Peripheral surgery for cervical dystonia and blepharospasm has been used for those patients who do not respond to botulinum toxin injections. There are various different options on offer. Myectomy refers to a surgical procedure in which a portion of an overactive muscle is removed. This was predominantly used in the treatment of blepharospasm, in which the muscle targeted was the orbicularis muscles or corrugator superficialis, until the advent of botulinum toxin injections. Peripheral denervation is also used most frequently in cervical dystonias. In this procedure the peripheral branch of the spinal accessory nerve to the sternomastoid muscle is sectioned and a posterior ramisectomy from C1 to C6 performed [34]. Improvements have been observed in 70–90% of patients although there is a risk of recurrence.

Physical treatment

In addition to medical treatment it is important to ensure that there is patient education and supportive care. Physical therapy, muscle relaxation techniques and well-fitting braces are helpful adjuncts to medical or surgical techniques and may improve posture and prevent contractures. However, braces tend to be tolerated poorly and are only really used for writer's cramp to enable the hand to be used more effectively and comfortably.

Conclusions

Dystonia remains a poorly understood disorder of movement that is inadequately recognised in day-to-day clinical practice. The condition can vary from a mild disorder to a disabling generalized condition, often with a genetic basis. Research addressing the genetics, prevalence and pathology of this heterogeneous condition has established the importance of recognition and awareness of this condition, although much more needs to be done. Effective treatment remains an unmet need in many, although botulinum toxin therapy and, more recently, deep brain stimulation surgery have been significant milestones of development.

References

1. Warner T. Dystonia. In: Birmingham Movement Disorders course. The Movement Disorder Society, 2008: 267–79.
2. Greene P. Medical and surgical therapy of idiopathic torsion dystonia. In: Kurlan R (ed.), Treatment of Movement Disorders. Philadelphia: JB Lippincott Co., 1995:153–181.
3. Jankovic J. Treatment of dystonia. Lancet Neurol 2006;5:864–72.
4. de Carvalho Aguiar P, Ozelius L. Classification and genetics of dystonia. Review. Lancet Neurol 2002;1:316–25.
5. Thyagarajan D. Dystonia: recent advances. J Clin Neurosci 1999; 6:1–8.
6. Geyer HL, Bressman SB. The diagnosis of dystonia. Lancet Neurol 2006; 5:780–790.
7. The Epidemiological Study of Dystonia in Europe (ESDE) Collaborative Group. A prevalence study of primary dystonia in eight European countries. J Neurol 2000; 247:787–792.
8. Matsumota S, Nishimura M, Sbiasski H, Kaji R. Epidemiology of primary dystonia in Japan; comparison with western countries. Mov Disord 2003; 18:1196–1198.
9. Sheehy MP, Marsden CD. Writer's cramp – a focal dystonia. Brain 1982; 105:461–80.
10. Blitzer A, Brin M, Fahn S, Lovelace RE. Clinical and laboratory characteristics of focal laryngeal dystonia: study in 110 cases. Laryngoscope 1988; 98:636–641.
11. Stojanovic M, Cvetkovic D, Kostic VS. A genetic study of idiopathic focal dystonias. J Neurol 1995; 242:508–511.
12. Fahn S, Bressman SB, Marsden CD. Classification of dystonia. Adv Neurol 1998; 78:1–10.
13. Gasser T. Inherited myoclonus dystonia syndrome. Adv Neurol 1998; 78:325–334.
14. Defazio G, Abbruzzese G, Livrea P, Berardelli A. Epidemiology of primary dystonia. Lancet Neurol 2004; 3:673–678.
15. Muller KS, Wenning GK, Seppi K. The prevalence of primary dystonia in the general community. Neurology 2002; 247:787–792.
16. Segawar M, Hosaka A, Miyagawa F, et al. Hereditary progressive dystonia with marked diurnal fluctuation. Adv Neurol 1976; 14:215-233.
17. Ichinose H, Ohye T, Takahiashi E, et al. Hereditary progressive dystonia with marked diurnal fluctuation caused by mutations in the GTP cyclohydrolase 1 gene. Nat Genet 1994; 8:236–242.

18. Lee LV, Pascasio FM, Fuentes FD, Viterbo GH. Torsion dystonia in Panay, Philippines. Adv Neurol 1976; 14:137–151.

19. Kupke KG, Lee L, Mueller U. Assignment of the X-linked torsion dystonia gene to Xq21 by linkage analysis. Neurology 1990; 40:1438–1442.

20. Brin MF, Jankovic J, Comella C, et al. Treatment of dystonia using botulinum toxin. In: Kurlan R (ed.), Treatment of Movement Disorders. Philadelphia: JB Lippincott Co., 1995; 183-246.

21. Lal S, Hoyte K, Kiely ME et al. Neuropharmacological investigations and treatment of spasmodic torticollis. Adv Neurol 1979; 24:335.

22. Burke RE, Fahn S, Marsden CD. Torsion dystonia: a double blind, prospective trial of high-dosage trihexyphenidil. Neurology 1986; 36:160–164.

23. Povlsen UJ, Pakkenberg H. effect of intravenous injection of biperiden and clonazepam in dystonia. Mov Disord 1990; 5:27.

24. Hoon AH, Freese PO, Reinhardt RH, et al. Age-dependent effects of trihexyphenidyl in extrapyramidal cerebral palsy. Pediatr Neurol 2001; 25:55–58.

25. Greene P, Shale H, Fahn S. Analysis of open-label trials in torsion dystonia using high dosages of anticholinergics and other drugs. Mov Disord 1988; 3:46.

26. Ziegler DK. Prolonged relief of dystonic movements with diazepam. Neurology 1981; 31:1457.

27. Walker R, Danisi F, Swope D, et al. Intrathecal baclofen for dystonia: benefits and complications during six years of experience. Mov Disord 2000;15:1242–1247.

28. Hou J-GG, Ondon W, Jankovic J. Intrathecal baclofen for dystonia. Mov Disord 2001; 16:1201–1202.

29. Naygaard T, Marsden CD, Fahn S. Dopa-responsive dystonia: long term treatment response and prognosis. Neurology 1991;41:174–181.

30. Greene P, Kange U, Fahn S, et al. Double blind, placebo controlled trial of botulinum toxin injections for the treatment of spasmodic torticollis. Neurology 1990; 40:1213.

31. Jost W, Blumel J, Grafe S. Botulinum toxin type A free of complexing proteins (XEOMIN) in focal dystonia. Drugs 2007; 67:668–683.

32. Adam OR, Jankovic J. Treatment of dystonia. Parkinsonism Relat Disord 2007;13 (suppl 3) :S362–368.

33. Krauss JK, Yianni J, Loher TJ, Aziz TZ. Deep brain stimulation for dystonia. J Clin Neurophysiol 2004; 21:18–30.

34. Bertrand C. Selective peripheral denervation for spasmodic torticollis: surgical technique, results and observations in 260 cases. Surg Neurol 1993; 40:96–103.

Chapter 4

Essential tremor

William G Ondo

Introduction

Essential tremor (ET) is a common neurological condition that is clinically diagnosed. Although several specific criteria exist, all require the presence of postural
or action tremor in the arms without any other neurological conditions to account
for such a tremor. Action tremor is identified in any scenario when those muscles
are volitionally used. In contrast, rest tremor, which is characteristic for Parkinson's
disease, occurs when the muscles are not volitionally engaged. For example, rest
tremor may occur when the arms are resting on the patient's legs or when dangling
while walking, while arm action tremor may occur when the patient is holding the
arms in front (postural tremor) or moving the hand back and forth between two
points (kinetic tremor). Intention tremor is also seen when moving between two
points; however, the amplitude increases when approaching the targeted points.
Intention tremor is usually seen in cerebellar pathology, such as multiple sclerosis.
In short, postural, kinetic and intention tremor are all subsets of action tremor.

Tremor isolated to other body parts but not involving the hands is generally considered to be "possible" ET. However, patients with "definite" ET often
have tremor in other body parts in addition to the hands. Most commonly
this includes the head and voice, but any part of the anatomy can be involved.
Usually the hands cause most of the disability.

In general, ET begins indolently at any age, often in childhood. The initial
amplitude is small whereas the frequency is relatively high (6–10 Hz). Over
decades the tremor amplitude increases whereas the frequency decreases. As it
is amplitude that correlates with functional disability, patients may have tremor
for many years before presenting to a physician. In older age, some ET patients
develop rest tremor and mild parkinsonian signs. The clinical classification
of these patients is debated. Some researchers allow mild parkinsonian signs
into the spectrum of ET, whereas others reclassify this phenotype as mixed
Parkinson's disease/ET.

Tremor subtypes and differential diagnosis

There are several different tremor sub-phenotypes (Figure 4.1) and their interrelationship is unclear. The tremor associated with dystonia is common and generates much debate. Dystonia is a patterned, involuntary movement discussed in Chapter 3. Often tremor and dystonia are seen together, and the tremor anatomy may be identical to or distant from the dystonia anatomy. Typically, the tremor seen with dystonia is irregular and jerky. The amplitude is usually smaller than with "pure" ET. About one-third of dystonia patients have some tremor. Some researchers consider tremor and dystonia as separate but related, whereas others feel that the tremor is just part of the dystonia, and refer to it as dystonic tremor rather than ET and dystonia.

Another tremor type that has some similarities to dystonia is task-specific tremor. These patients demonstrate no or minimal observable tremor with arm posture or even simple movements. However, when they perform a specific task, such as writing, typing, playing a musical instrument, applying make-up or golf putting, they will develop marked oscillation. Over time this may generalize to less specific actions; for example, tremor may initially start when writing the cursive letter "e", while later tremor is seen with all cursive writing but not when drawing a straight line or drawing a picture, then script writing has tremor, and later still general drawing is affected. Finally other hand actions may be affected and the patient may even have some modest postural tremor seen when their hands are held in front. This also progresses to a rest tremor in some cases.

Orthostatic tremor is an interesting, very-low-amplitude, high-frequency (typically 14 Hz) tremor in the legs present only when the patient is standing. It can also occur in the arms if patients stand on their arms or apply similar pressure to their arms. It is an elusive diagnosis because the tremor is often not visible and patients actually present with balance difficulty that improves with ambulation. They usually do not complain of tremor at all, but are very apprehensive about standing still and usually stand with a wide stance with the arms abducted to improve their subjective balance. Despite this, formal balance testing is normal and they do not fall [1]. The diagnosis is made by palpating the calves while the patient is standing. Usually a vibration can be felt, although it may not be palpable for a few minutes after standing. Surface electromyogram (EMG) can confirm a 14 Hz tremor. Orthostatic tremor is an important differential diagnosis in someone complaining of balance problems.

Fragile X-associated tremor ataxia disorder (FXTAS) is a recently defined disorder that may be confused with, and used to be diagnosed as, ET [2]. The tremor is usually seen only after the age of 50. The kinetic tremor is usually

Tremor subtypes

	Frequency (Hz)	Anatomy/Quality	Associated features	Treatment
Enhanced physiological tremor	8–12	Distal hands Voice	Occurs with stress or physical activity	None β-blockers as needed
Essential tremor	4–12	Any Arms > head > voice	Mild ataxia Hearing loss Restless legs syndrome	β-blocker Primidone Topiramate Benzodiazepines Botulinum toxin VIM DBS
Dystonic tremor	3–12	Hands/neck Jerky Variably rhythmic	Dystonia	β-blocker Benzodiazepines Anticholinergics Botulinum toxin Primidone VIM DBS
Task-specific tremor	3–8	Specific anatomy associated with task, usually hand	None	Responds poorly to medications β-blockers Botulinum toxin VIM DBS
Orthostatic tremor	14	Often palpable in legs only on standing	Marked subjective balance difficulty while standing but not walking	Medications often help transiently Clonazepam Gabapentin Phenobarbital Topiramate
FXTAS	2–8	Kinetic > postural	Ataxia, parkinsonism, dementia Family history of fragile X in grandchildren	Same as ET but may be less responsive
Cerebellar outflow tremor	2–6	Proximal and distal, truncal Large amplitude Very disabling	Secondary to head trauma, space-occupying lesions, multiple sclerosis	Poorly responsive to medications Benzodiazepines, weights, VIM DBS
Parkinson's disease	3–6	Rest tremor: when muscle is not volitionally contracted	Parkinsonism	Dopaminergic medications, zonisamide VIM or STN DBS

Figure 4.1 Tremor subtypes. DBS, deep brain stimulation; ET, essential tremor; FXTAS, fragile X-associated tremor ataxia disorder; STN, subthalamic nucleus; VIM, ventralis intermedius nucleus.

much larger than the postural tremor. Often patients have modest ataxia, and parkinsonism and dementia can also occur. Magnetic resonance imaging (MRI) often shows T2-weighted lesions in the cerebellar outflow tracts. Genetic testing demonstrating an intermittent CGG repeat length (50–200 trinucelotide repeats) on the fragile X gene is diagnostic. Although the same gene is affected in clinical fragile X syndrome (learning disability in childhood), the clinical phenotype, protein transcription and translation of the gene are markedly different.

Although not part of any diagnostic criteria, there may be moderate balance difficulties, augmented age-dependent hearing loss and possibly mild cognitive deficits in "regular" ET [3,4]. These other symptoms and signs are generally mild, although balance difficulties may be problematic in elderly people and confuse the diagnosis with Parkinson's disease.

Physical examination and clinical evaluation

Patients are often examined with their arms forward, arms in the "wing-beating position" with elbows extended and hands near the nose, during finger-to-nose touching maneuvers, and while writing their name and drawing spirals. Tremor should be specifically sought in the voice ("aaaaaaaa"), head (while turning the head in all directions) and legs. The patient should be observed for signs of Parkinson's disease (muscle rigidity and slowness/smallness of movement). Some young-onset Parkinson's disease patients present with unilateral action tremor rather than rest tremor. The presence of dystonia (patterned, sustained muscle movements such as neck rotation, wrist flexion while writing and foot inversion while walking) should be evaluated. In general, electrophysiological measurement with EMG (measuring muscle contractions) or accelerometry (measuring the actual movement in space) do not add to the assessment of ET. In fact, the presence of typical ET probably does not justify any other evaluation, with the possible exception of thyroid tests.

Epidemiology and neuropathology

Essential tremor affects between 0.1% and 6.0% of the population depending on the inclusion criteria, probably 1–2% by the most widely accepted definitions. Men and women are equally affected. About 60% of individuals presenting for evaluation have a family history of tremor, and, in fact, ET is often called "familial" or "benign familial" tremor. One gene and several genetic linkage sites have been identified but there are no commercially available tests for them. Given the wide distribution of tremor, it is likely that multiple genes will eventually be discovered.

Experimental imaging studies of the brain (positron emission tomography or PET) in patients with ET show increased activity in the cerebellum and probably in the inferior olive in the medulla. Some studies also shows increased thalamic activity, and cell recording during operations for ET show neurons firing in tandem with the tremor. Several other modalities, including single photon emission computed tomography (SPECT), confirm this increased activity. Normally available tests, such as MRI, are unremarkable in ET.

Pathological evaluation of the brain does not show consistent or unique abnormalities, but two different patterns have emerged [5]. Some patients have findings consistent with mild Parkinson's disease, including Lewy bodies. The second pattern is modest cerebellar cell loss with "torpedo" inclusions, a non specific finding associated with cell stress. Many ET patients have demonstrated no clear brain pathology at autopsy. In general, it is suspected that hypersynchronization of intrinsic pacemaker cells within these areas precipitates the motor oscillation of tremor but there is no clear evidence to support this.

Treatment

In general, the treatment literature for ET is less stringent than for some other neurological conditions, and the use of only a few treatments are supported by "class A" data [6]. Furthermore, the literature is hampered by the lack of a single accepted rating scale, so comparisons are difficult. The treatment of ET can be separated into oral medications, botulinum toxin injections and surgical interventions (Figure 4.2).

Arguably, the most consistent tremorlytic agent is ethanol. Tremor suppression usually occurs within 20 min and lasts for 3–5 h. Often it is followed by a rebound tremor augmentation. The equivalent of one drink appears adequate. The use and abuse of alcohol are probably not increased in ET patients, although this is debated. Other less intoxicating alcohols are currently being studied for ET [7].

β-blockers are a well-established and well-studied ET treatment. Although comparative data are minimal, noncardioselective β-blockers, such as propranolol, nadolol and sotalol, probably confer a stronger tremorlytic response. Propranolol is conventionally used because of its well-supported efficacy, low cost and dosing flexibility. The half-life of propranolol is approximately 5 hours; however, a long-acting preparation is available. A direct dose–response relationship is seen with β-blockers and they can be used on an as-needed basis. In most studies, propranolol reduces tremor by about 50%. It is generally started at 10 or 20 mg up to three times a day, titrating each dose by 10–20 mg until either there is a satisfactory improvement or adverse events stop the titration. Doses of up to 320 mg/day are sometimes used. Once a dose has been established the patient can be switched to a long-acting preparation if desired. Nadolol has been less well studied but offers the advantage of a longer half-life. The dose ranges from 40 mg to 160 mg/day.

Medications for essential tremor

Treatment	Total daily dose (mg) and number of doses	Comment	Adverse events
β-blockers: propranolol, nadolol	Propranolol 10–320 two to three times daily Nadolol 20–160 once daily	Dose-dependent effect. Can be used as required	Fatigue, hypotension, bradycardia, masked hypoglycemia
Primidone	25–300 two to three times daily	AEs usually with first dose Pretreatment with 3 days of 30 mg phenobarbital reduces AEs	Dizziness, nausea, ataxia
Topiramate	25–400	Dose-dependent effect	Cognitive worsening, tingling, altered taste, weight loss, kidney stones, acute vision change
Gabapentin/ pregabalin	Gabapentin 300–3200 three times daily Pregabalin 75–300 twice daily	Variable efficacy	Weight gain, edema, dizziness, sleepiness
Zonisamide	50–200 twice daily	Variable efficacy. Also helps PD tremor	Similar to topiramate, but usually milder
Benzodiazepines	As tolerated	May help with anxiety and ET	Sedation, cognitive slowing, dizziness, dependency
Leviteracetam	500–2000 twice daily	Mild efficacy	Minimal AEs
Botulinum toxin	Variable	Injected into muscles for tremor of distal arm, head, jaw	With training very safe Local weakness, bruise
VIM DBS		Reserved for severe tremor, best for hand tremor	Any CNS surgical complication, dysarthria, balance

Figure 4.2 Medications for essential tremor. AEs, adverse events; CNS, central nervous system; DBS, deep brain stimulation; ET, essential tremor; PD, Parkinson's disease; VIM, ventralis intermedius nucleus.

The noncardioselective β-blockers such as atenolol have also demonstrated efficacy for ET, but the effect size is somewhat smaller. Adverse events (AEs) of β blockers are well established and include bradycardia, hypotension, erectile dysfunction, general fatigue, depression, exacerbation of reactive airway disease and masking of hypoglycemia. In a geriatric population the general sense of fatigue is the most common problematic event. It should be noted that these drugs are not absolutely contraindicated in diabetes or congestive heart failure.

Primidone is the other long-established treatment for ET. Studies establish efficacy at doses ranging from 50 mg three times daily to 250 mg three times daily. The drug was originally created for epilepsy and is metabolized to phenobarbital, which also modestly improves tremor and possesses a very long half-life. Most studies of primidone demonstrate a 50–75% tremor reduction; however, comparative studies against propranolol have never demonstrated any efficacy difference between the two.

In my experience, this drug works best with "classic" sinusoidal ET that is not associated with dystonia. It is also more "hit or miss". AEs include dizziness, ataxia, nausea and malaise. If they occur they are almost always experienced with the first dose, and can be severe. After a few days they usually subside and the drug is subsequently well tolerated. To minimize this first pill affect, the initial dose should be 25 mg at night. We usually start with 30 mg phenobarbital at night for three nights, which autoinduces the metabolism of primidone and further reduces the chance of AEs.

Topiramate is another antiepileptic medication that can improve ET. A large multicenter trial confirmed its tremorlytic effect at doses from 25 mg twice daily up to 200 mg twice daily [8]. A moderate dose–response relationship was seen. The medication has multiple possible mechanisms of action and seems to help all tremor types, including parkinsonian tremor. AEs are common and most commonly include paresthesia, altered sense of taste, cognitive slowing, especially dysphasia and weight loss. More serious AEs include kidney stones, reported in about 1% of chronic users and resulting from urine alkylation, and ciliary edema, resulting in acute bilateral blurred vision. I usually begin at 12.5 mg twice daily and titrate up to 200 mg twice daily or until satisfactory improvement occurs or AEs intervene.

The use of other pharmacological agents is supported by far less research. Gabapentin has had mixed results in three controlled trials. The drug is generally well tolerated and has been studied in doses up to 1200 mg three times daily. Benzodiazepines have long been used to treat ET; however, only alprazolam improved tremor in controlled trials. The medications may be most useful in treating tremor specifically triggered by stress. Clozapine is the prototypical "atypical" antipsychotic. A single controlled trial demonstrated efficacy against ET. It has also separately demonstrated efficacy in motor features of Parkinson's disease. The drug carries a risk of agranulocytosis and requires weekly complete blood count monitoring. Therefore, it is seldom used for ET. Other drugs reported to help ET include the carbonic anhydrase inhibitor acetazolamide, the calcium channel blockers nimodipine and flunarizine, and clonidine.

There has been little study of polypharmacy for ET. Several open-label studies have supported the concurrent use of primidone and β-blockers. Anecdotally, polypharmacy with drugs from different classes seems to confer additional benefit.

Botulinum toxin A has over 200 medical uses supported in the literature, The drug inhibits acetylcholine from being released from the nerve terminal by lysing one of the required SNARE proteins. Therefore, there is no acetylcholine-triggered calcium influx into the muscle, and the muscle stops contracting. Typically this lasts for 3–4 months before the nerve terminal regenerates. Multiple trials of both arm tremor and head tremor have variably demonstrated efficacy of botulinum toxin, with more consistently robust results seen in head tremor [9]. There is great utility for botulinum toxin in arm tremor that primarily involves the wrists, task-specific tremors such as writing tremor, head tremor and jaw tremor. The treatment has essentially no systemic AEs, but can cause local weakness. The other limiting factor is cost, which is usually not covered by insurance.

When tremor amplitude becomes very large, pharmacological agents are seldom satisfactory. In these patients, and those refractory to other agents, the use of deep brain stimulation (DBS) into the ventralis intermedius (VIM) thalamus is justified. This procedure is now nearly 15 years old and has dramatically helped thousands of ET patients. A stereotactic frame is placed and the VIM thalamus located. The device is actually tested in the operating room to ensure appropriate placement. The patients then undergo brief general anesthesia and the pulse generator is implanted under the clavicle or abdomen. Most patients are discharged the next day. They later return for adjustments of several electrical parameters to optimize response.

The exact mechanism of action is debated, but the procedure mimics the effects of a lesion to the same area, rather than stimulating that area as the name suggests. One large study comparing DBS with thalamotomy (burning a lesion into the thalamus) found that they were equally effective but that DBS had a better safety profile [10]. Although formal comparisons of DBS with best medical management have not been done, there is little doubt that this procedure offers the most robust treatment effect size in patients with severe tremor. Surgical AEs are usually minimal. During adjustments, patients most commonly experience paresthesia, dysarthria or balance difficulties. These usually resolve with further adjustments but are much more common when the devices are implanted bilaterally. It is usual to implant unilaterally at first and wait at least 3 months before a second procedure. The benefit:risk ratio is larger for the first side than for the additional second side; however, the decision to implant bilaterally must be individualized.

References

1. Fung VS, Sauner D, Day BL. A dissociation between subjective and objective unsteadiness in primary orthostatic tremor. Brain 2001; 124:322–330.
2. Leehey MA, Munhoz RP, Lang AE, et al. The fragile X premutation presenting as essential tremor. Arch Neurol 2003; 60:117–121.
3. Ondo W, Vuong K, Sutton L, Jankovic J. Assessment of hearing loss in essential tremor. Neurology 2001; 58(suppl 3):A433–434.
4. Singer C, Sanchez-Ramos J, Weiner WJ. Gait abnormality in essential tremor. Mov Disord 1994; 9:193–196.
5. Louis ED, Vonsattel JP. The emerging neuropathology of essential tremor. Mov Disord 2008; 23:174–182.
6. Zesiewicz TA, Elble R, Louis ED, et al. Practice parameter: therapies for essential tremor: report of the Quality Standards Subcommittee of the American Academy of Neurology. Neurology 2005; 64:2008–2020.
7. Bushara KO, Goldstein SR, Grimes GJ Jr, et al. Pilot trial of 1-octanol in essential tremor. Neurology 2004; 62:122–124.
8. Ondo WG, Jankovic J, Connor GS, et al. Topiramate in essential tremor: a double-blind, placebo-controlled trial. Neurology 2006; 66:672–677.
9. Simpson DM, Blitzer A, Brashear A, et al. Assessment: botulinum neurotoxin for the treatment of movement disorders (an evidence-based review): report of the Therapeutics and Technology Assessment Subcommittee of the American Academy of Neurology. Neurology 2008; 70:1699-1706.
10. Schuurman P, Bosch A, Merkus P. A comparison of continuous thalamic stimulation and thalamotomy for suppression of severe tremor. N Engl J Med 2000; 342:461-468.

Chapter 5

Restless legs syndrome

William G Ondo

Restless legs syndrome

Restless legs syndrome (RLS) is currently defined as [1]:

- An urge to move the limbs with or without sensations
- Worsening at rest
- Improving with activity
- Worsening in the evening or night.

The diagnosis of RLS is exclusively based on these four criteria, all of which are required to make the diagnosis. A validated diagnostic phone interview [2], rating scales [3] and quality-of-life scales [4] have all been developed based on these features.

Patients, however, seldom quote the RLS inclusion criteria at presentation, and often have difficulty describing the sensory component of their RLS. The descriptions are quite varied and tend to be suggestive and education dependent. The sensation is always unpleasant but not traditionally painful in most cases. It is usually deep within the legs. In one study, the most common terms used, in descending order of frequency, included: "need to move", "crawling", "tingling", "restless", "cramping", "creeping", "pulling", "painful", "electric", "tension", "discomfort" and "itching" [5]. Patients usually deny any "burning" or "pins and needles" sensations, commonly experienced in neuropathies or nerve entrapments, although neuropathic pain and RLS can coexist. Arm involvement is common but generally only occurs after many years of leg involvement. The face and torso should not be involved in RLS.

Essentially all patients report that walking produces transient symptomatic improvement, although some employ stationary bike riding, kicking or any other volitional movement. Other therapeutic techniques reported by patients include rubbing or pressure, stretching and hot water. Symptom relief strategies all increase sensory stimulation to the legs and are generally alerting. This can be a problematic strategy when sleep is desired.

Other clinical features typical for RLS include the tendency for symptoms to gradually worsen with age, improvement with dopaminergic treatments, a positive family history of RLS and periodic limb movements of sleep (PLMS). It should be noted, however, that PLMS are not part of the definition of RLS.

Periodic limb movements of sleep

PLMS is defined by the Association of Sleep Disorders as "periodic episodes of repetitive and highly stereotyped limb movements that occur during sleep". They are reported in standard polysomnography but may be adequately described by a bed partner. PLMS can occur simultaneously in both legs, alternate between legs or occur unilaterally. The duration of movement is typically between 1.5 and 2.5 seconds and varies in intensity from slight extension of the great toe to a triple flexion response (hip, knee and ankle all flexing). Patients frequently demonstrate a movement periodicity of between 20 and 40 seconds, although wider ranges of frequencies have been reported. Movements are most pronounced in stage I and stage II sleep, where they are often accompanied by K-complexes and increases in pulse and blood pressure.

The incidence of PLMS in the general population increases with age and is very high in elderly people, but very low in children. The largest single study in RLS patients, employing a cut-off of five PLMS/hour, reported that 81% of patients showed pathological PLMS [6]. The prevalence increased to 87% if two nights were recorded. Although PLMS accompanies most cases of RLS, many patients with PLMS do not have RLS. In contrast, most people with RLS do have PLMS. The exact relationship between the two phenotypes is unclear but some feel that they are highly related.

RLS in children

RLS in children can be difficult to diagnose. Although some children report classic RLS symptoms that meet inclusion criteria, others complain of "growing pains", and some appear to present with an attention deficit hyperactivity disorder (ADHD) phenotype. The official NIH RLS diagnostic criteria in children are vague and have never been validated. These criteria emphasize supportive criteria such as a family history of RLS and sleep disturbances and the presence of PLMS, which is uncommon in control children [1].

The potential relationship between RLS and ADHD is very interesting. Children diagnosed with ADHD often have PLMS, and may meet criteria for RLS [7]. Children with ADHD also have a higher prevalence of a parent with RLS [8] and children diagnosed with PLMS often have ADHD. Both ADHD and RLS are also treated with dopaminergics and both are associated with low iron levels in some studies.

Differential diagnosis in restless legs syndrome

Disorder	Comment
Neurological disorders with "urge to move"	
Neuroleptic-induced akathisia	Looks like severe RLS but affects the whole body, not just the limbs. Less circadian and less relief from movement. Entire body rocking often seen. Associated with dopamine antagonists
Hypotensive akathisia	Feeling of restlessness that may be localized in legs, brought on by sitting still; should not occur while lying down but might be relieved by movement; occurs in patients with orthostatic hypotension
Volitional movements, foot tapping, leg rocking	Occurs in individuals who fidget, especially when bored or anxious, but usually do not experience associated sensory symptoms, discomfort or conscious urge to move; symptoms do not bother the person, usually lack a circadian pattern; more of a type of psychic restlessness; fewer sleep disturbances; very common
Painful legs and moving toes	Feet involved more; movement truly involuntary; no circadian pattern; usually have continuous slow writhing
Isolated leg stereotype	Fast (>3 Hz) rhythmic plantar flexion/dorsiflexion movements oscillating around ankle, but sometimes involving additional leg anatomy. Usually a tremor phenotype but not considered a true tremor. It is easily suppressed and is almost always seen only while sitting. The condition is common, not considered pathological, may be an alerting activity, and overlaps with foot tapping/leg rocking
Orthostatic tremor	Fine leg tremor that is manifest by a sense of poor balance while standing, but not while walking; therefore patients cannot stand still but need to walk There are no symptoms while sitting or lying down. No circadian pattern
Disorders without "urge to move"	
Nocturnal leg cramps	Leg cramps or "charley horse" cramps can come on at night and are relieved with stretching or walking; no urge to move; experienced as a usually painful muscular contraction, often involving the calf muscles, unlike RLS sensations; sudden onset, short duration, usually palpable contractions
Arthritis, lower limb	Discomfort centered more in joints, may not have prominent circadian pattern as seen in RLS, increased symptoms during movement, does not respond to dopaminergics, usually no periodic limb movements of sleep
Positional discomfort	Often comes on with prolonged sitting or lying in the same position but usually relieved by a simple change in position, unlike RLS, which often returns when change of position, movement or walking is not continued; no circadian pattern
Vascular disorders	
Vascular claudication	Pain in the legs, Usually worse with walking/movement and usually relieved by prolonging rest; often best in a lying position; no urge to move; no circadian pattern; usually no sleep disturbances

Figure 5.1 Differential diagnosis in restless leg syndrome (RLS). Modified from Benes et al. [9] Continued overleaf.

Differential diagnosis in restless legs syndrome (*continued*)	
Varicose veins	May have discomfort in legs; some relief with massage or inactivity
Pain disorders	
Myelopathy, radiculopathy	Dysesthesias and pain in the legs, frequently one sided, often radicular; atrophic changes of musculature; no urge to move the legs; symptoms can be initiated by sitting and lying and improve by movement; does not respond to dopaminergic therapy
Painful peripheral neuropathy	Sensory symptoms commonly reported as numbness, burning and pain; more superficial, no urge to move, complete and persistent relief not obtained while walking or during sustained movement
Isolated leg pain	Undiagnosed leg pain/ache in the muscle may be seen without other explanation; examination and evaluation normal; is often worse at night and may improve with movement but there is no true urge to move
Congestive heart failure	Night-time pain in the lower limbs spreading to the lumbosacral area can occur and causes sleep disturbances; no urge to move; attributed to nocturnal engorgement of the lumbar veins causing transient lumbar stenosis
Fibromyalgia	Multiple, alternating, multiform complaints in muscle groups and joints; sometimes leg accentuated but mostly whole body affected; frequent sleep disorders, no circadian pattern, no relief by movement
Sleep-related disorders	
Periodic limb movements of sleep	Diagnosis made by sleep laboratory assessment, positive response to dopaminergic therapy, no urge to move or dysesthesias while awake; sleep disturbance and complaints of daytime fatigue and sleepiness may be present
Hypnic jerks	Involuntary muscle (myoclonic) twitch that occurs while falling asleep, described as an electric shock or falling sensation, which can cause movements of legs and arms; occurs once or twice per night; common.

Figure 5.1 continued.

Diagnostic evaluation

In most cases, only a simple evaluation is justified for clinically typical RLS. Serum ferritin, and possibly iron-binding saturation should be measured in order to assess if serum iron deficiency is present and electrolytes for renal failure should be obtained. Nerve conduction velocities (NCVs) and an electromyogram (EMG) may be performed in cases without a family history of RLS, atypical presentations (such as sensations beginning in the feet or superficial pain), in cases that have a predisposition for neuropathy (ie, diabetes), or when physical symptoms and signs are consistent with a peripheral neuropathy. Polysomnographic evaluation is usually reserved for patients in whom the diagnosis is in doubt, in cases where

PLMS is suspected to be severe and results in arousals, or if other sleep disorders, such as sleep apnea, are suspected. A careful history and physical examination are generally sufficient to make a diagnosis of RLS.

In most cases, the diagnosis is relatively easy; however, some conditions can be confused with RLS. Akathisia is most similar. Patients have an inner sense of restlessness accompanied by an intense desire to move and often rock in place. The restlessness is usually generalized, but may be most prominent in the legs. These individuals do not typically complain of any limb paresthesia. Importantly, it is usually associated with the use of dopamine antagonists. Nocturnal leg cramps are a common, multifactorial, disorder manifested by paroxysmal, disorganized spasms that usually involve the feet or calf muscles. The presentation is quite different from RLS, but patients may initially describe their RLS symptoms simply as "night cramps", which can lead to misdiagnosis if a more extensive history is not taken. Other conditions are summarized in Figure 5.1.

Epidemiology

Historically, epidemiological studies of RLS were limited by the subjective nature of the disease, the lack of standardized diagnostic criteria, and the indolent onset of the condition. Most studies from Europe and the USA report that about 10% of all people have RLS and 2–3% have RLS with a severity that warrants chronic pharmacological therapy. Women are affected more than men by a 2:1 ratio. The largest epidemiological study of RLS involved more than 23,000 persons from five countries [10]. Similar to smaller reports, 9.6% of all people met criteria for RLS. In general, northern European countries demonstrated higher prevalence compared with Mediterranean countries. The vast majority of these individuals were not previously diagnosed, despite frequently reporting symptoms to their physicians.

RLS can occur in all ethnic backgrounds; however, it seems that white people are most affected. Asian populations report lower prevalences, usually 1–3%. People of African descent have never been specifically studied but anecdotally African–Americans only rarely present with RLS. It is unclear whether this represents a true lower prevalence, or rather differences in referral patterns.

Genetics

In roughly 60% of cases, a family history of RLS can be found, although this is often not initially reported by the patient [5]. Twin studies also show a very high concordance rate. Most pedigrees suggest an autosomal dominant pattern, although an autosomal recessive pattern with a very high carrier rate is possible. A younger age of onset is associated with a greater likelihood of familial disease.

To date four genes that confer risk for RLS have been identified in population-based studies [11,12]. Several of these seem to be involved with embryological development of the spine and limbs. Six other genetic loci have been identified in individual family linkage studies but no specific allele or mutation has been identified. Therefore, there is currently no genetic test for RLS.

Pathophysiology

Pathological research suggests that the pathophysiology of RLS involves central nervous system (CNS) iron homeostatic dysregulation. Cerebrospinal fluid (CSF) ferritin is lower in RLS cases [13], and specially sequenced magnetic resonance imaging (MRI) studies and ultrasonography show reduced iron stores in the striatum, red nucleus and substantia nigra [14,15]. Most importantly, pathological data from autopsied brains of people who had RLS show reduced ferritin staining and iron staining, and increased transferrin stains, but also reduced transferrin receptors. Research also demonstrates reduced Thy-1 expression, which is regulated by iron levels [16]. The reduced transferrin receptor finding is important because globally reduced iron stores would normally upregulate transferrin receptors. Therefore it appears that primary RLS has reduced intra cellular iron indices secondary to a perturbation of homeostatic mechanisms that regulate iron influx and/or efflux from the cell. This may involve iron regulatory protein-type 1 (IRP-1) [17]. It should be noted that serum iron indices do not correlate well with CSF iron.

CNS dopaminergic systems are strongly implicated by the dramatic response to dopaminergic medications. That said, there is little pathophysiological data to suggest that reduced dopamine causes RLS. Substantia nigra dopaminergic cells are not reduced in number, nor are there markers associated with neurodegenerative diseases, such as tau or α-synuclein abnormalities [18,19]. Pathologically, dopamine is relatively normal or elevated and dopamine type 2 receptors were reduced in the striatum. Dopamine imaging studies of the striatum have been very inconsistent and difficult to interpret.

The relationship between the observed iron-deplete pathology and response to dopaminergics is not known. One theory suggests that the reduced iron decreases Thy-1 activity, which is needed for the release of monoamines, such as dopamine, into the nerve synapse.

Another remaining puzzle is the identification of the specific anatomy culpable for RLS. Involvement of the seldom-studied diencephalospinal dopaminergic tract, originating from the A11–A14 nuclei, might explain some RLS features. It is involved in anti-nociception (pain control), is near circadian control centers and is dopaminergic, and its spinal trajectory would explain why the legs are involved more than arms. An animal model with A11 lesions demonstrated increased activity that improved with dopaminergic medications. Anatomical and physiological assessments of the spinal cord in RLS are lacking in humans.

Secondary RLS

Several other neurological and medical conditions are associated with higher rates of RLS than would be expected and are sometimes referred to as "secondary RLS". The most common causes of secondary RLS include renal failure, iron deficiency, neuropathy, myelinopathy, pregnancy, and possibly Parkinson's disease and essential tremor. There is also some evidence to support an association of RLS with some genetic ataxias, fibromyalgia, rheumatological diseases and migraines. A variety of other associations have been suggested but these are at best tenuous.

As discussed, reduced CNS iron is implicated in all cases of RLS. It is intuitive to suggest that reduced body stores of iron could also result in low CNS intracellular iron and cause RLS symptoms. Numerous reports have associated low serum ferritin levels with RLS. This seems most robust in patients with no family history of RLS and in those with an older age of onset. These groups, however, generally represent the same population because there is a very strong correlation between a younger age of RLS onset and the presence of a family history of RLS. Serum ferritin is the best indicator of low iron stores and the only serum measure to consistently correlate with RLS. Anemia has not been independently associated with RLS and is not an adequate screen for iron deficiency. Oral iron supplementation is recommended when ferritin is low, but only open-label trials support this strategy.

Of the common associations, neuropathy is the most controversial. In summary, most studies that have evaluated RLS populations have found higher rates of neuropathy than would be expected; however, most population studies of neuropathy patients have not found higher rates of RLS. Axonal, rather than demyelinating, neuropathies may be associated more with RLS. Traumatic spinal cord lesions, neoplastic spinal lesions, demyelinating or post-infectious lesions, and syringomyelia can all precipitate RLS and PLMS.

Uremia secondary to renal failure is strongly associated with RLS symptoms. Numerous series report a 20–57% prevalence of RLS in renal dialysis patients; however, only a minority of uremic patients volunteer RLS symptoms unless specifically queried [20]. Studies evaluating specific risk factors for RLS in the uremic population have been inconclusive. The prevalence of RLS in mild-to-moderate renal failure that does not require dialysis is unknown. The RLS seen in dialysis patients is often severe and associated with worse leg movements.

Both RLS and PLMS have also been associated with increased mortality in the dialysis population.

Overall, dialysis does not improve RLS. However, patients who undergo a successful kidney transplantation usually experience dramatic improvement in RLS within days to weeks. The degree of symptom alleviation appears to correlate with improved kidney function.

The development of RLS during pregnancy has long been recognized. Manconi et al. [21] recently evaluated risk factors for RLS in 606 pregnancies.

Drug	Amount per dose (mg)	Duration effect (hours)	Comment
Medications used to treat restless legs syndrome (RLS)			
Dopaminergics: immediate effect, considered first line therapy			
Levodopa	100–250	2-6	Approved in Europe, fast onset, can use prn, highest augmentation rates
Pramipexole	0.125–1	5–12	Approved, commonly used, slower onset but longer duration
Ropinirole	0.25–4	4–8	Approved, slow-release preparations available
Pergolide	0.125–1	6–14	Well studied but seldom used due to risk of cardiac valve fibrosis and other possible ergot adverse events (AEs)
Cabergoline	0.25–2	>24	Longest acting but may have same AEs as other ergot dopamine agonists
Rotigotine	0.5–6	24	Patch preparation well studied and effective in RLS
Bromocriptine	5–20	4–6	Rarely used in RLS
Opioids: numerous opioids used			
Methadone	2–15	8–12	Latency to benefit
Hydrocodone	5–10	4–10	Faster acting, shorter duration
Epilepsy drugs			
Gabapentin	300–1200	4–8	May help painful component of RLS
Pregabalin	50–200	6–12	Trials under way but almost no published data
Gabapentin enacarbil	600–12,000	8–16	Gabapentin prodrug with better absorption and pK profile; well studied and effective
Benzodiazepine			
Clonazepam	0.5–2		More beneficial for sleep than RLS, can be used in combination with other RLS medications
Iron supplementation			
Oral iron	>50	?	No specific iron salt superior, titrate up as tolerated. Ferritin will only modestly increase
Intravenous iron dextran	1000	?	Usually not repeated before 3 months, several days latency to benefit, long-term safety unknown. Patients with "normal" serum ferritin equally responsive

Figure 5.2 Medications used to treat restless legs syndrome (RLS). Prn, pro re nata (as needed).

They reported that 26% of these women suffered from RLS, usually in the last trimester. The authors could find no significant differences in most risk factors; however, hemoglobin was significantly lower in the RLS group, and plasma iron tended to be lower, compared with those with no RLS.

Parkinson's disease and RLS respond to similar medications and both have PLMS; however, their pathologies are markedly different. Studies evaluating RLS in the Parkinson's disease population usually show that 20% of Parkinson's disease patients have clinical RLS. In most cases the Parkinson's disease presents first, and the RLS is relatively mild and does not contribute much to the morbidity of Parkinson's disease. Importantly, there is no evidence that RLS evolves into Parkinson's disease.

About 30% of patients presenting with ET also have RLS [22]. In contrast to these other conditions these patients often have a family history of both conditions, suggesting a distinct disease with an ET/RLS phenotype.

Finally, several medications are known to exacerbate existing RLS or possibly precipitate RLS themselves. The most notable of these include antihistamines, dopamine antagonists, including many anti-nausea medications, mirtazapine, and possibly tricyclic antidepressants and serotonin reuptake inhibitors. Antihistamines, found in many non-prescription preparations, most consistently worsen RLS and PLMS. There effect is immediate whereas dopamine antagonist-induced exacerbation may be gradual.

Treatment

Multiple medications have demonstrated outstanding efficacy; however, all are felt to provide only symptomatic relief, rather than "curative" effect. Therefore, treatment should be initiated only when the benefits are felt to justify any potential adverse events and costs. Treatment decisions also need to consider the chronicity and general progressive course of RLS. Over time, both dosing and medication changes are required to maximize the benefit and minimize the risk of tolerance and adverse events. Medications used to treat RLS are summarized in Figure 5.2 and described below.

Dopamine antagonists

Dopamine agonists (DAs) are clearly the best investigated and probably the most effective treatments for RLS. The improvement is immediate and often very dramatic. Multiple large placebo-controlled trials support the efficacy of pramipexole, ropinirole, pergolide, transdermal rotigotine and levodopa. Fewer data support cabergoline, bromocriptine and lisuride. No evidence favors any particular DA, but several DAs have proved superior to levodopa. The DAs improve all aspects of RLS, including PLMS. Sleep generally improves; however, there is no overt change in sleep architecture. Interestingly, lower doses may improve sleep more than higher doses.

DAs are best administered 1–2 hours before the onset of symptoms. If symptoms occur earlier in the evening this may necessitate multiple doses to control symptoms throughout the night. Individualized timing of these drugs is critical to their success. This is in contrast to the approved dosing timing, usually 1–3 hours before bed. The effect is immediate, so titration can be fairly rapid. The smallest possible dose is initiated and increased until satisfactory improvement is achieved. The adverse events of DA are different in RLS and Parkinson's disease; RLS patients do not become psychotic, develop dyskinesia or demonstrate hypotension. The sedative properties are generally not a problem in RLS but nausea, edema and impulse control disorders can occur.

The long-term use of DAs for RLS can be more problematic. Patients can develop tolerance and dopamine-induced augmentation. Augmentation is defined by an earlier phase shift of symptom onset, an increased intensity of symptoms, increased anatomical involvement or less relief with movement. It was first noted and is still most problematic with levodopa, which has the shortest half-life of any dopaminergic medication. Augmentation correlates with greater doses of drug and a positive family history of RLS. The mechanisms behind augmentation are not known, however, and it is reported with all dopamine agonists but not with other classes of medications. There are no data supporting any strategy to prevent augmentation or indicating how to manage it when it occurs. Earlier dose administration is usually employed but this may eventually fail.

Augmentation improves about a week after DA withdrawal so drug holidays and alternative treatment with opioids can be considered.

Opioids

Opioid medications, also known as narcotics, have long been known to successfully treat RLS. Open-label trials consistently demonstrate good initial and long-term results, with no difficulty with tolerance, dependence or addiction. There are, however, only minimal controlled data, and no prospective comparative data. μ-Opioid agonists, which are usually more potent analgesics, are probably most effective. Meperidine and codeine are the least effective. Opioids are used as second-line therapy, usually methadone, which is a long-acting μ-specific agonist. Interestingly, there are data suggesting that the clinical benefit is independent of their general analgesic properties. The use of dopamine antagonists will negate an opioid's beneficial effect on RLS but not on pain.

Gabapentin

Gabapentin is an antiepileptic with affinity for the $\alpha_2\delta$ subunit of the voltage-dependent calcium channel, and is used to treat many neurological conditions. The drug increases slow-wave (deep) sleep but reduces PLMS less than DAs. Gabapentin is fairly innocuous but may cause dizziness, sedation and weight gain. Dosing should be individualized and begin about 2 hours before symptom onset. Two similar medications, pregabalin and gabapentin enacarbil, are undergoing large, multicenter trials, and may be approved for RLS in the near future.

Other treatments

Despite their past widespread use, there are few data to support the use of benzodiazepines for RLS. In the opinion of most experts, benzodiazepines do help facilitate sleep but seldom improve RLS cardinal features. These can be used successfully in mild cases of RLS and as adjunct therapy for residual insomnia.

Oral iron supplementation may modestly and gradually improve RLS. Gastrointestinal side effects, especially constipation, can limit use. In contrast, the administration of intravenous iron can dramatically increase serum ferritin levels and an open-label study of intravenous iron demonstrated robust efficacy [23]. Iron dextran, which is known to cause allergic reactions, may work best. After a small test dose, 1 g can be administered over 4 h in an infusion center. Improvement usually occurs after a few days and lasts for weeks to several months. Our lack of knowledge about the safety of chronic high-dose intravenous iron relegates this to a third-line treatment.

Numerous other agents, including other antiepileptic medications, clonidine, baclofen, tramadol and magnesium, have been reported to help RLS but suffer from limited data and cannot be recommended as either first- or second-line therapy. Sensory stimuli, such as hot water, pain infliction and inflatable compression hose, are often used by patients.

References

1. Allen RP, Picchietti D, Hening WA, et al. Restless legs syndrome: diagnostic criteria, special considerations, and epidemiology. A report from the restless legs syndrome diagnosis and epidemiology workshop at the National Institutes of Health. Sleep Med 2003; 4:101–119.

2. Hening WA, Allen RP, Thanner S, et al. The Johns Hopkins telephone diagnostic interview for the restless legs syndrome: preliminary investigation for validation in a multi-center patient and control population. Sleep Med 2003; 4:137–141.

3. Walters AS, LeBrocq C, Dhar A, et al. Validation of the International Restless Legs Syndrome Study Group rating scale for restless legs syndrome. Sleep Med 2003;4:121–132.

4. Atkinson MJ, Allen RP, DuChane J, et al. Validation of the Restless Legs Syndrome Quality of Life Instrument (RLS-QLI): findings of a consortium of national experts and the RLS Foundation. Qual Life Res 2004; 13:679–693.

5. Ondo W, Jankovic J. Restless legs syndrome: clinicoetiologic correlates. Neurology 1996; 47:1435–1441.
6. Montplaisir J, Boucher S, Poirier G, et al. Clinical, polysomnographic, and genetic characteristics of restless legs syndrome: a study of 133 patients diagnosed with new standard criteria. Mov Disord 1997; 12:61–65.
7. Chervin RD, Archbold KH, Dillon JE, et al. Associations between symptoms of inattention, hyperactivity, restless legs, and periodic leg movements. Sleep 2002; 25:213–218.
8. Picchietti DL, Underwood DJ, Farris WA, et al. Further studies on periodic limb movement disorder and restless legs syndrome in children with attention-deficit hyperactivity disorder. Mov Disord 1999;14:1000–1007.
9. Benes H, Walters A, Allen R, et al. Definition of restless legs syndrome, how to diagnose it, and how to differentiate it from RLS mimics. Mov Disord 2007; 22(suppl 18):S401–408.
10. Hening W, Walters AS, Allen RP, et al. Impact, diagnosis and treatment of restless legs syndrome (RLS) in a primary care population: the REST (RLS epidemiology, symptoms, and treatment) primary care study. Sleep Med 2004; 5:237–246.
11. Winkelmann J, Schormair B, Lichtner P, et al. Genome-wide association study of restless legs syndrome identifies common variants in three genomic regions. Nat Genet 2007; 39:1000–1006.
12. Schormair B, Kemlink D, Roeske D, et al. PTPRD (protein tyrosine phospatase receptor type delta) is associated with restless legs syndrome. Nature Genetics 2008; 40:946-948.
13. Earley CJ, Connor JR, Beard JL, et al. Abnormalities in CSF concentrations of ferritin and transferrin in restless legs syndrome. Neurology 2000; 54:1698–1700.
14. Allen RP, Barker PB, Wehrl F, et al. MRI measurement of brain iron in patients with restless legs syndrome. Neurology 2001; 56:263–265.
15. Schmidauer C, Sojer M, Stocckner H, et al. Brain parenchyma sonography differentiates RLS patients from normal controls and patients with Parkinson's disease. Mov Disord 2005; 20(suppl 10):S43.
16. Wang X, Wiesinger J, Beard J, et al. Thy1 expression in the brain is affected by iron and is decreased in restless legs syndrome. J Neurol Sci 2004; 220:59–66.
17. Connor JR, Wang XS, Patton SM, et al. Decreased transferrin receptor expression by neuromelanin cells in restless legs syndrome. Neurology 2004;62:1563–1567.
18. Pittock SJ, Parrett T, Adler CH, et al. Neuropathology of primary restless leg syndrome: absence of specific tau- and alpha-synuclein pathology. Mov Disord 2004; 19:695–699.
19. Connor JR, Boyer PJ, Menzies SL, et al. Neuropathological examination suggests impaired brain iron acquisition in restless legs syndrome. Neurology 2003; 61:304–309.
20. Chow K Hui D. Restless legs syndrome and renal failure. In: Ondo WG (ed.), Restless Legs Syndrome. New York: Informa Healthcare, 2006.
21. Manconi M, Govoni V, Cesnik E, et al. Epidemiology of restless legs syndrome in a population of 606 pregnant women. Sleep 2003;26:A300–301.
22. Ondo W. The association of restless legs syndrome and essential tremor. Mov Disord 2005; 20:S160.
23. Earley CJ, Heckler D, Allen RP. The treatment of restless legs syndrome with intravenous iron dextran. Sleep Med 2004; 5:231–235.

Chapter 6

Other movement disorders

William G Ondo

Drug-induced movement disorders

Drug-induced movement disorders remain a common and under-recognized problem. Blockade of the dopaminergic system results in multiple syndromes and will be the main focus of this discussion. These syndromes are often referred to as extrapyramidal side effects (EPSE) and include tardive dyskinesia, acute dystonic reactions, akathisia, drug-induced parkinsonism and neuroleptic malignant syndrome (Figure 6.1). Serotonin syndrome and drug-induced tremor are also briefly discussed.

Tardive dyskinesia

Tardive dyskinesia (TD) is the most prevalent problematic EPSE. The general descriptor "dyskinesia" is used because the phenotype is variable. Most commonly, patients demonstrate an oral–buccal–lingual stereotype. A stereotype is repetitive and patterned, but not oscillatory enough to be a tremor. The movements are partially or totally suppressed by volitional activity. For example, some patients have tongue movements that are visible when the tongue is relaxed inside the mouth but this will stop when the patient extrudes the tongue. These movements may be palpable and audible (causing sounds like gum being chewed) but even opening the mouth can cause them to subside. The feet are the next most frequently involved anatomical area but any area can be involved. Other phenotypes include tics (episodic movements out of a normal background), tremor, chorea, dystonia and pain. The pain is characteristically difficult to describe but is consistently in the midline (mouth and pelvis), and poorly responsive to opioid medications. Patients with tardive pain may or may not have concurrent movements.

TD may occur at any point during or just after treatment with dopamine antagonists. The total risk is cumulative. As a rule 5% per year incidence is a good estimate. It is somewhat lower with newer agents that have relatively less dopamine receptor affinity [1]. Withdrawal dyskinesia almost always occurs within 1 year of stopping dopamine antagonists, usually within a few months.

Drug-induced movement disorders

	Phenotype	Risk factors	Prognosis	Treatment
Parkinsonism	Identical to PD but may be more symmetrical and faster tremor	Old age, baseline parkinsonism	Resolves with drug discontinuation unless underlying parkinsonism; may develop mild TD	Drug withdrawal Amantadine, anticholinergics, dopaminergic medications
Rabbit syndrome	4–6 Hz large-amplitude mouth tremor	Female	Variable	Anticholinergics, amantadine
Acute dystonic reaction	Upward eye deviation Neck extension	Young age, male	Resolves in several days	Antihistamines, anticholinergics, benzodiazepines (usually only one dose required) Diphenhydramine 50 mg most commonly used
Tardive dyskinesia	Variable Usually mouth, tongue, jaw repetitive smooth movements that lessen with volitional action	Old age, female, diabetes, organic brain disorder	Persistent but may gradually lessen over years. Withdrawal TD has a better prognosis	Tetrabenazine Vitamin B$_6$ Vitamin E Botulinum toxin Benzodiazepines GP$_i$ deep brain stimulation
Acute akathisia	Inner body: need to move; pacing, rocking	Possible iron deficiency	Improves with drug withdrawal	Drug withdrawal
Tardive akathisia	Inner body: need to move, pacing, rocking	?	Variable, may persist for years	Benzodiazepines, β-blockers
Neuroleptic malignant syndrome	Rigidity, autonomic instability (fever), altered mental status	?	25% mortality rate Improves over months	Dopamine agonists, dantroline, supportive care

Figure 6.1 Drug-induced movement disorders. GP$_i$, globus pallidus interna; PD, Parkinson's disease; TD, tardive dyskinesia.

As other medicines are often substituted for the true offending agents, withdrawal dyskinesia is often incorrectly blamed on the new drug. Withdrawal dyskinesia usually has a better long-term prognosis.

Risk factors for TD consistently include older age and female sex. For example, an 80-year-old woman probably has a 20–25% per year incidence of TD while on these medications. Other possible risk factors include diabetes mellitus, organic brain injury, affective disorders and depot drug preparations. As would be expected, the potency of the dopamine blocker is a risk factor. Many nausea medications are potent causes of TD. Although formal data are lacking, metoclopramide may be the most culpable overall agent due to its long-term use. Medications that raise the risk of TD (dopamine receptor affinity) are listed in Figure 6.2.

The overall prognosis for TD is for it to remain static or very gradually improve. Removal of the offending agent actually initially worsens TD, or precipitates it in the case of withdrawal dyskinesia. The same medicines that cause the condition therefore partially suppress it, although maintaining the drug as a "treatment" is not a good strategy for most patients because long-term prognosis worsens as a function of how long the patient stays on a medication while having symptoms. Therefore, it is recommended that the drug is discontinued at the first sign of TD if at all possible.

Risk of extrapyramidal side effects in drugs that block dopamine receptors		
High risk	**Medium risk**	**Low risk**
Haloperidol	Promazine	Quetiapine
Fluphenazine	Olanzapine	Clozapine
Metoclopramide	Ziprasidone	Promethazine
Prochlorperazine	Aripiprazole	Trimethobenzamide
Risperidone		Domperidonea
Pimozide		
Droperidol		
Thioridazine		
Trifluperazine		

Figure 6.2 Risk of extrapyramidal side effects in drugs that block dopamine receptors.

Treatment of TD may be difficult. The best overall medication is tetrabenazine [2]. This is a "dopamine depletory" that reduces the release of dopamine, and other neurotransmitters to a lesser degree. In reducing dopamine it can cause parkinsonism, akathisia and depression. The drug is titrated to effect in two or three times daily dosing. The usual daily dose ranges from 25 mg to 100 mg.

Other treatments are much less consistent. Vitamin B_6 (pyridoxine) 300 mg, branched-chain amino acids (leucine, isoleucine, valine) and vitamin E (α-tocopherol) have been shown in controlled trials to have efficacy in TD.

However, only one group has reported efficacy for branched-chain amino acids and vitamin B_6, and most vitamin E studies have not shown any benefit [3,4]. Benzodiazepines, acetylcholinesterase inhibitors (developed for Alzheimer's disease) and other muscle relaxant medicines may occasionally help. Botulinum injections may help but this depends on the specific anatomy. For example, tongue movement is not very amenable to botulinum injections. Finally deep brain stimulation of the globus pallidus internus, a site targeted for both Parkinson's disease and dystonia, may help in severe cases of tardive dystonia.

Acute dystonic reaction

Acute dystonic reaction is a benign, mostly self-limiting, but dramatic movement usually seen in children or young adults 2–5 days after starting a dopamine blocker. Typically, there is sudden ocular deviation (eyes rolled upward) and extensor dystonia (neck and even back extension). Mental status is preserved but parents often think that a seizure is occurring and usually seek immediate attention. It is thought that this reaction occurs during a short window when dopamine receptor levels and endogenous dopamine release are both increased. Dystonic reactions probably occur in 1–5% of patients who start dopamine blockers, although epidemiological data vary markedly.

The condition consistently responds to antihistamines, such as diphenhydramine (usual dose 50 mg i.v). Oral antihistamines, anticholinergics and benzodiazepines are also effective. Typically, after treatment, the condition will not recur, and it is not necessary to discontinue the offending agent. This potential side effect should be discussed with parents before initiation of dopamine blockers because, unless they are told that it is a once-only event, they will almost never continue the drug if an acute dystonic reaction occurs.

Drug-induced parkinsonism

A whole range of medications may cause parkinsonism, the most notable being typical dopamine receptor-blocking antipsychotic agents such as thioridazine, chlorpromazine and haloperidol. These may cause acute akinetic or dystonic crises along with an oculogyric crisis. Drug-induced parkinsonism (DIP) is the most common cause of secondary parkinsonism and may be misdiagnosed as Parkinson's disease, because their clinical features overlap considerably, with the presence of rigidity, bradykinesia, tremor and gait disturbance, and may even be asymmetric. Figure 6.3 gives a list of medications reported to cause DIP. There is some evidence that patients who develop DIP may have subclinical Lewy body Parkinson's disease, which may be unmasked by dopamine-blocking agents. The effects of dopamine-blocking agents may be prolonged, and DIP may take up to 9 months to disappear. The incidence of DIP is estimated to be 15–40% in patients receiving neuroleptics, and its prevalence increases with age. A DaT scan may help in differentiating DIP from Parkinson's disease because most DIP is postsynaptic and as such is likely to show a normal DaT scan uptake.

Clinically, DIP may be more symmetrical and have a slightly faster tremor than idiopathic Parkinson's disease; however, a true clinical distinction is impossible. In fact, on the basis of imaging and pathology studies, about 30% of DIP cases have evidence of idiopathic Parkinson's disease [5,6]. The medications probably accelerated the clinical presentation but these patients would have eventually developed idiopathic Parkinson's disease.

Treatment consists of withdrawal of the offending medication. If drug withdrawal is impractical, patients are given the lowest possible dose or are changed to a new atypical agent, such as clozapine or quetiapine. Anticholinergics may be of some benefit; the role of levodopa treatment is unknown.

DIP should resolve upon discontinuation of the offending medication; however, this may not occur for up to 3 months. If the agent cannot be discontinued, or at least reduced, amantadine is anecdotally effective. Other dopaminergic medications can be used effectively although the combination

Drugs reported to cause or precipitate parkinsonism

Drugs linked to dopamine metabolism
Inhibitors of dopamine synthesis or precursors of a false neurotransmitter:
- α-Methyl-*p*-tyrosine
- α-Methyldopa

Drugs that affect dopamine neuronal level:
Lithium
Presynaptic dopamine storage inhibitors:
- Reserpine
- Tetrabenazine

Postsynaptic D2-receptor blocking:
- Tetrabenazine
- Flunarizine
- Amoxapine

Atypical neuroleptics:
- Risperidone
- Olanzapine

Benzamides:
- Metoclopramide

γ-Aminobutyric acid (GABA) agonists:
- Sodium valproate

Calcium-channel blockers:
- Cinnarizine
- Flunarizine

Neuroleptics:
- Phenothiazines
  - prochlorperazine
  - amitriptyline
  - thioridazine
  - promethazine
  - fluphenazine
  - mesoridazine
  - trifluoperazine
  - chlorpromazine
  - thiethylperazine
  - perphenazine
- Butyrophenones
  - haloperidol
- Thioxanthenes
  - thiothixene
- Benzamides
  - metoclopramide
- Dihydroindolone
  - molindone
- Dibenzoxazepine
  - loxapine

Figure 6.3 Drugs reported to cause or precipitate parkinsonism.

of dopamine agonists and antagonists is less than desirable. Anticholinergics are also used effectively for DIP, but they are not helpful for the prevention or treatment of TD.

Neuroleptic malignant syndrome

Neuroleptic malignant syndrome is defined by the presence of hyperthermia and possibly other autonomic lability, altered mental status and rigidity, often with muscle breakdown and elevated serum creatine phosphokinase (CPK) levels. The traditional mortality rate is 30% although this may have become lessened in recent years. Neuroleptic malignant syndrome can occur at any time during a course of dopamine-blocking drugs with an incidence of about 0.1%. The pathophysiology is almost entirely unknown.

Treatment of neuroleptic malignant syndrome includes hospitalization with supportive care. The muscle breakdown can cause rhabdomyolysis and subsequent renal failure. This and respiratory failure can lead to death. Traditional treatments include dantroline (a muscle relaxant that blocks intracellular calcium influx) and dopamine agonists. Bromocriptine has traditionally been used but longer-acting dopamine agonists such as pramipexole, ropinirole and cabergoline can also be used.

Akathisia

Akathisia is an inner sense of restlessness and a need to move. Typically patients will rock in a chair or pace back and forth in a room and look very anxious. They have difficulty verbalizing their actual sensations so these indirect signs are important. The condition differs from restless legs syndrome in that the entire body is involved, as opposed to isolated limb involvement; patients pace, instead of slowly twisting their legs, and there is a less marked circadian pattern, although symptoms of akathisia may be worse at night.

Most cases of akathisia are acute, meaning that they occur while taking the offending dopaminergic antagonist. These will rapidly improve when the drug is stopped, or reduced. Benzodiazepines and β-blockers such as nadolol or propranolol are used but there are almost no published data.

Serotonin syndrome

Serotonin syndrome is variably defined and somewhat more vague than side effects of dopaminergic blockade. It is usually associated with serotonin reuptake inhibitors (SSRIs) and may be seen when these drugs are used in monotherapy or combined with other medications. Monoamine oxide (MAO) A inhibitors used as antidepressants, as well as possibly MAO-B inhibitors used in Parkinson's disease (rasagiline, selegiline), and triptan medications used for migraine headaches may also increase serotonin. Interestingly meperidine is probably the most likely drug to cause serotonin syndrome. A well-known death from meperidine and an MAO-A inhibitor in the USA actually resulted in major changes in medical training regulations [7].

Symptoms and signs of serotonin syndrome include tremor, anxiety/agitation and diarrhea. Additional symptoms can include flushing, tachycardia, insomnia, fever, mydriasis and hyperreflexia. Severity varies tremendously.

Mild cases require no specific treatment. Severe cases with autonomic symptoms and altered mental status should be hospitalized and monitored. Aside from drug withdrawal, treatments include β-blockers and benzodiazepines. The fever is usually refractory to typical antipyretic medications.

Drug-induced action tremor

Many drugs can accentuate the normal physiological tremor that is present in all people (Figure 6.4). The tremor is seen with the hands placed outward and with motion. It is relatively fast and of low amplitude, and may have a jerky quality. The voice and head may also be involved. If treatment is necessary, the offending agent can be discontinued or reduced and/or β-blockers such as propranolol or nadolol can be used.

Drugs that may commonly cause action tremor	
β-agonist inhalers	Steroids
Stimulants, ie methylphenidate	Lithium[a]
Serotonin reuptake inhibitors	Valproate[a]
Buproprion	Amiodarone
Theophylline	

Figure 6.4 Drugs that may commonly cause action tremor. [a]Usually causes some tremor.

Tics and Tourette's syndrome

Tourette's syndrome (also known as Gilles de la Tourette's syndrome) is somewhat arbitrarily defined [8]. The most widely recognized criteria for diagnosis require:

- two or more motor tics and one vocal tic
- onset under the age of 21
- a duration of more than 1 year
- no other explanation for the tics.

A tic is an "unvoluntary" movement or sound out of a normal background. Tics that occur but do not meet criteria for Tourette's syndrome are variably

Secondary causes of tics

Idiopathic
Tourette's syndrome, chronic multiple motor tic disorder, phonic/vocal tic disorder, chronic single tic disorder, transient tic disorder, nonspecific tic disorder

Genetic disease
Huntington's disease, torsional dystonia, neuroacanthocytosis

Infectious
Encephalitis, Creutzfeldt–Jakob disease, Sydenham's chorea

Drugs
Methylphenidate, amphetamines, cocaine, levodopa, anticonvulsants, antipsychotics

Toxins
Carbon monoxide

Other
Static encephalopathy, trauma, ischemia, chromosomal disorders, neurocutaneous syndromes

Figure 6.5 Secondary causes of tics.

codified but there are no data to suggest any intrinsic difference between Tourette's syndrome and multifocal motor tic disorder or other similar conditions. Most tics are idiopathic but many other disorders have tics as part of their phenotype (Figure 6.5).

Tics are partially suppressible, but suppression is often associated with an increased urge or tension. Tics are suggestible, often occurring when they are discussed. Tics also have a sensory or premonitory component, often just preceding the actual movement. This combination of suppressibility, suggestibility and sensory component differentiates tics from myoclonus, dystonia or other movements.

Tics are common and affect 1–10% of all children, with boys being more represented. They can first occur at any age with a mean age at onset of 6. As a rule, tic severity waxes and wanes until the late teens and then improves. Meaningful tics persisting past the third decade are uncommon. Tics are relatively mild in most cases and most children with mild tics are never diagnosed or seek medical attention. However, tics can be very severe, resulting in complete isolation from society or even bodily injury. Tics can involve any part of the body but eye blinking, shoulder shrugging and rotation, and head tilting are the most common. Although coprolalia (using inappropriate "bad" language) is synonymous with Tourette's syndrome, it occurs in about only 10% of cases. The most common vocal tics are guttural "ggpp" sounds and sniffing. In fact, children with Tourette's syndrome are commonly misdiagnosed with allergies secondary to sniffing tics and tic sensations in their throat. Tourette's syndrome is often accompanied by other neuropsychiatric syndromes such as obsessive–compulsive disorder and attention deficit disorder, but these do not define the condition.

There are four treatment classes for tics: behavioral therapy, pharmacotherapy, botulinum toxin and surgery. In all cases one must remember that tics wax and wane, the pathophysiology is not well understood, treatments are considered symptomatic and tics usually improve over the years. In all cases side effects must be balanced against improvement.

Although desirable, behavioral treatments have not demonstrated consistent efficacy. The most common is habit reversal training, where patients try to replace the tic with an unnoticed movement such as clenching their fist. Anxiety-relieving techniques, such as biofeedback, cognitive therapy and exposure desensitization, are also occasionally tried.

The mainstay of pharmacotherapy remains dopamine antagonists (neuroleptics) (Figure 6.6). I prefer fluphenazine but pimozide and haloperidol are commonly used. Formal data are lacking but newer "atypical" antipsychotics, with fewer dopamine antagonist affinities, are probably not as effective. Dopamine antagonists typically reduce tics by 50–75% from baseline in a dose-dependent manner. Side effects can be problematic. Sedation, fatigue and reduced motivation are the most common. Akathisia, weight gain, heat intolerance and acute dystonic reaction can occur. TD, although possible, is rare in children. Other useful medications include tetrabenazine, a dopamine-depleting agent; topiramate, a seizure medication; and clonidine, an α_1 antagonist. Numerous other medications have been reported to help in some cases. Immunomodulation with plasmapheresis has been advocated but controlled trials were negative. In all cases these drugs provide symptomatic treatment. The choice of drug is based on anticipated side effects and comorbid conditions, and frequently involves trial and error.

Botulinum toxin inhibits muscle contraction by blocking the release of acetylcholine in the neuromuscular junction. Although now commonly known as a cosmetic treatment, it was developed, and commonly used, to treat a variety of hyperkinetic movement disorders. Botulinum toxin can effectively treat tics in certain anatomies, mostly the upper face (eye blinking, forehead contractions, paranasal movements) and neck (head pulling and rotation, and shoulder shrugging). Therefore the treatment is reserved for patients with problematic tics in these areas. Interestingly the treatment usually improves the premonitory sensation, not just the movement. It often results in complete cessation of

Treatment options for tics

Class	Relative efficacy[a]	Drug	Daily dose (mg)	Specific side effects	Class side effects
Neuroleptics (dopamine antagonists)	+++	Fluphenazine	1–12		Sedation, fatigue, weight gain, akathisia, acute dystonic reactions, tardive dyskinesia
		Pimozide	2–15	QT prolongation	
		Haloperidol	1–15		
		Thioridazine		QT prolongation	
		Risperidone	0.5–12	Weight gain	
		Ziprasidone		No weight gain	
		Olanzapine	2.5–30	Weight gain	
Dopamine depletory (VMAT-2 inhibitor)	+++	Tetrabenazine	12.5–150		Sedation, sleep disturbance, akathisia, acute dystonic reaction, depression
α_2-blockers	++	Clonidine	0.05–0.9 Patch TTS1-3		Sedation, fatigue, hypotension
		Guanfacine	1–9		
Benzodiazepines (traditionally clonazepam but others can be used)	+	Clonazepam	0.25–9		Sedation, reduced concentration/cognition, personality changes
Dopamine agonists	+	Pramipexole	0.25–3.0		Nausea, hypotension, edema, impulsivity
		Ropinirole	0.25–12.0		
		Pergolide	0.1–1.5	Cardiac valvulopathy	
Seizure medications	++	Topiramate	25–600		Decreased memory, paresthesia, altered taste, weight loss, renal stones
Nicotine	+	Nicotine	Various patch/pill/gum preparation		Marked nausea

Figure 6.6 Treatment options for tics. [a]Based on experience of the author. VMAT-2, vesicular monoamine transporter type 2.

the injected tic but some patients subsequently manifest tics in different areas after the injections.

Psychosurgery has a long and checkered history. Recently, deep brain stimulation has been used for severe cases of tics. Various targets are used including the globus pallidus internus, the anterior limb of internal capsule and several areas of the thalamus. Results in open-label series have ranged from modest to dramatic and life changing. Psychosurgery is of course reserved for the most severe and refractory cases.

Chorea, ballismus and athetosis

Chorea, ballismus and athetosis are irregular, nonpatterned writhing or "dance-like" movements. Ballismus has a more proximal origin (shoulder and hip) and is slower than chorea. Athetosis is slower and more writhing in nature. The distinction among the three remains because different diseases are associated with them. Physiologically they are fairly similar.

Chorea

Chorea is the most common of the three and has a large differential diagnosis, especially if chorea is one of many abnormalities. A large number of rare inborn errors of metabolism may include chorea as part of their broader phenotype. Figure 6.7 lists relatively common conditions in which chorea is usually the primary feature. A comprehensive list of conditions where chorea has been reported runs into the hundreds.

The most common chorea is Huntington's disease, manifested by chorea, dementia and psychiatric abnormalities, bulbar symptoms and gait disturbance [9]. The phenotype is age dependent. Young-onset Huntington's disease (Westphal variant) presents with parkinsonism, tremor, seizures and rapid cognitive decline. Older-onset patients may present only with chorea, whereas middle-aged patients usually present with personality changes, which are followed by chorea.

The condition is an autosomal dominant disease associated with CAG triplet repeats on chromosome 4. A younger age of onset is partially predicted by a longer length of the repeat. Repeats of more than 80 usually present in childhood, repeats in the 40s usually present in midlife, and the variant with 28–32 repeats is a borderline positive gene with variable penetrance.

Symptomatic treatment of chorea includes the use of tetrabenazine, neuroleptics, amantadine, benzodiazepines, and several epilepsy medications including valproate, leviteracetam, carbamazepine, phenytoin and topiramate. In the author's experience epilepsy medications are seldom effective.

Differential diagnosis of chorea

Category	Disease	Comment	Treatment
Genetic	Huntington's disease	Accompanied by dementia, psychiatric, bulbar and balance symptoms. Young onset has parkinsonism and seizures; AD	TBZ, amantadine
	Huntington disease-like type 2	Seen in black people of South African descent. Younger onset has a parkinsonian/dementia phenotype; AD	TBZ
	Dentatorubro-pallidoluysian atrophy (DRPLA)	Also called Haw River syndrome, Japan; frequently seen African–Americans; MRI shows atrophy and white matter changes; AD	
	Neuroacanthocytosis	Onset 20–40, T2-weighted MRI lesions in caudate, various subtypes, positive acanthocyte smears, AR > AR > X linked	
	Hereditary benign chorea	Classic form has thyroid and pulmonary disease. Young onset. Caused by mutation in thyroid transcription factor-1, AD	
Autoimmune/ infectious	Sydenham's chorea	Often delayed after group A streptococcal infections; elevated antistreptolysin; other neuropsychiatric symptoms, especially obsessive–compulsive disorder; MRI normal	Antibiotics, TBZ, prednisone
	Numerous infectious encephalopathies	Chorea appears concurrent with or after encephalopathy; MRI may show transient T2-weighted striatal hyperintensities; improves over months	Underlying infection
	Antiphospholipid syndrome	Some have anti-cardiolipin antibodies, may have headache, thrombosis, other features of lupus	Autoimmune therapy
	Paraneoplastic	Anti-collapsin response-mediator protein (CRMP-5) not included in some "paraneoplastic panels". Usually small cell lung carcinoma	Underlying neoplasm
Miscellaneous	Hyperthyroidism	Also myoclonus, tremor, psychiatric changes	Underlying condition
	Post-cardiac surgery	Also known as "post-pump" syndrome in children	Mixed results with TBZ and steroids
	Chorea gravidarum	Women often had post-infectious chorea in childhood	Delivery
	Static encephalopathy	"Cerebral palsy" ± MRI changes; chorea phenotype associated with relatively normal cognition. Chorea may be delayed by decades – "delayed-onset dyskinesia"	
	Kernicterus	Chorea, athetosis, dystonia, reduced extraocular movements, deafness	Light therapy in perinatal period
	Vascular chorea	Diagnosis of exclusion, usually diffuse small vessel disease except for hemiballism	
Medications	Estrogen, anabolic steroids, amphetamine-type medications, ie methylphenidate, lithium, epilepsy medications, dopaminergics in Parkinson's disease		

Figure 6.7 Differential diagnosis of chorea. AD, autosomal dominant; AR, autosomal recessive; MRI, magnetic resonance imaging; TBZ, tetrabenazine.

Hemiballismus

Hemiballismus classically follows a lesion (ischemic stroke, hemorrhagic stroke or neoplasm) in or adjacent to the subthalamic nucleus (Figure 6.8a). It often occurs several days after the acute event, which in some cases is not otherwise symptomatic. It may be very severe, completely disabling the patient secondary to large-amplitude arm and/or leg movements. It is not suppressible but may be worse with attempted volitional movements. The prognosis is for gradual improvement over months to years, but there is little change in the short term.

Hemichorea–hemiballismus is an interesting phenomenon seen during hyperglycemia, commonly before and heralding the diagnosis of diabetes mellitus. There is usually a characteristic magnetic resonance imaging (MRI) signal (Figure 6.8), which is diagnostic. With proper glycemic control, the chorea improves over days to weeks in most cases. The MRI lesion also improves.

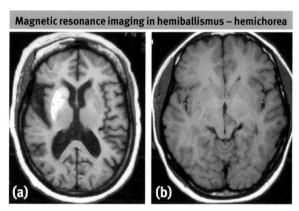

Magnetic resonance imaging in hemiballismus – hemichorea

(a) (b)

Figure 6.8 Magnetic resonance imaging (MRI) in hemiballism–hemichorea. (a) T1-weighted MRI pattern in diabetic hemiballism/hemichorea. (b) T1-weighted MRI showing arteriovenous malformation encompassing the subthalamic nucleus.

In refractory cases, tetrabenazine is very effective, often at lower doses than required for other choreas and hemiballismus [10].

Treatment of hemiballismus can be difficult. Tetrabenazine, also used for chorea, is probably the best agent. Neuroleptics (such as haloperidol), amantadine, benzodiazepines and several seizure medications such as leviteracetam, valproate and topiramate are occasionally effective. Large doses of botulinum toxin can help but the proximal muscles of the arm and leg generally respond less well. Stereotactic surgery (ablative or deep brain stimulation) targeting the outflow tract of the subthalamic nucleus is used in refractory and long-standing cases.

Athetosis

Athetosis is slow chorea. It is often associated with increased muscle tone, similar to dystonia, but, unlike in dystonia, the movements are not well-patterned. Frequently the entire trunk is involved. Static encephalopathy (cerebral palsy) is by far the most common etiology. Kernicterus (perinatal hyperbilirubinemia) was once a common cause but is seldom seen today. A pseudo-athetosis of the limbs can be seen with severe neuropathy or other de-afferentation, as a result of reduced proprioception. The treatment of athetosis is poor. Similar medications to those for chorea and hemiballismus are used but the response is usually unsatisfactory.

Myoclonus

Myoclonus means quick jerk-like muscle movements. These are usually very rapid (<0.25 seconds), simple movements. Myoclonus is classified in several different ways. Clinically it is divided by anatomy (generalized, axial, multifocal or focal), whether or not it is rhythmic, and whether it is spontaneous or induced by action (movement) or reflex (in response to visual, tactile or audio stimuli). It is sometimes classified by its site of origin within the nervous system because sophisticated electrophysiological investigations can sometimes discriminate these, in which case it is divided into cortical, subcortical (reticular/brain-stem), spinal and peripheral. Myoclonus is also defined by its exact etiology when this is known. "Hypoxic myoclonus" is the best example of this. Some myoclonus types, such as hiccoughs (singultus) and sleep starts (body jerks as one is falling asleep), are not considered to be pathological.

As with chorea, a complete list of conditions that have ever been associated with myoclonus is very lengthy. A list of relatively common conditions is presented in Figure 6.9.

Severe myoclonus can be refractory to many medications. Often treating the underlying abnormality in secondary causes will help. The myoclonic epilepsies, especially juvenile myoclonic epilepsy, respond well to valproate or other seizure medications. In general, benzodiazepines, traditionally clonazepam, are most commonly used. Seizure medications, baclofen or tetrabenazine are variably employed. Botulinum toxin can be very effective for focal myoclonus, especially hemifacial spasm.

Ataxia

Ataxia means the breakdown of smooth movement. It is commonly manifest by gait difficulties, arm coordination problems, speech (not language) breakdown and tremor. The ataxic gait is wide based (legs spread apart) and looks jerky and uncoordinated, and often slow due to the poor balance. Patients are unable to tandem walk on a line. Abnormal arm movement signs include past pointing and dysdiadochokinesis.

Causes of myoclonus

Physiological
Hypnic jerks (sleep starts) – typically while falling asleep
Hiccough – myoclonus of the diaphragm
Exercise/anxiety – often seen with tremor

Epileptic
Juvenile myoclonic epilepsy – characteristic electroencephalogram changes
Progressive myoclonus epilepsy (Unverricht–Lundborg syndrome)
Myoclonic astatic epilepsy (Lennox–Gastaut syndrome)
Infantile spasms
Fragment of epileptic discharges (partial continuous epilepsy)

Idiopathic
Familial essential myoclonus (also known as myoclonus dystonia, alcohol responsive,
dystonia with lightning jerk)
Epsilon-sarcoglycan gene mutations
Sporadic idiopathic myoclonus

Symptomatic
Lance–Adams syndrome (postanoxic action myoclonus)
Electric shock
Heat stroke
Blunt head trauma
Any central nervous syndrome lesion: tumor, hemorrhage, stroke, abscess
Neurodegenerative movement disorders:
- Wilson's disease – caused by copper accumulation
- PANK-2 – caused by iron accumulation
- multiple system atrophy
- Huntington's disease
- corticobasal degeneration – usually present
- progressive supranuclear palsy
- dentatorubro-pallidolusian atrophy
- Parkinson's disease – uncommon

Dementias:
- Creutzfeldt–Jakob disease – usually present
- dementia with Lewy bodies
- Alzheimer's dementia

Infectious diseases:
- herpes encephalitis – usually present
- subacute sclerosis panencephalitis – "hung" slow myoclonus
- AIDS
- Whipple's disease
- any viral encephalitis

Metabolic:
- hepatic failure –classically negative myoclonus, asterixis
- renal failure
- hypoglycemia
- hyperglycemia, especially nonketotic hyperglycemia
- hyponatremia

Figure 6.9 Causes of myoclonus. Continued overleaf.

Causes of myoclonus (continued)

Toxic:
- various heavy metals
- bisthmuth
- serotonin syndrome
- dopaminergics

Miscellaneous:
- celiac disease
- mitochondrial encephalopathies
- numerous inborn errors of metabolism: often associated with ataxia
- palatal myoclonus:
  - idiopathic
  - secondary to brain-stem lesions
- hemifacial spasm – spontaneous contraction of facial muscles; usually caused by compression of the facial nerve
- other peripheral nerve injuries
- startle syndromes (reflex myoclonus):
  - hyperekplexia
  - jumping Frenchman, Latah, Rajon Cajon

Figure 6.9 *continued*.

Patients will miss an object that they are trying to touch by overshooting or under-shooting the depth. The rhythmicity and smoothness of repetitive movements such as hand pronation/supination break down. Speech is classically scanning, with a loss of prosidy (rhythm). It may speed up and then slow down. Volume also varies. Tremor is an intention–related type, such that the amplitude increases as the hand approaches its goal. Head tremor in this setting is called titubation. Patients may have only some of these features. For example, chronic alcohol-induced ataxia usually involves gait whereas lesions in the midbrain cause mostly tremor and arm ataxia.

Many varied etiologies can result in ataxia (Figure 6.10). Classification is usually based on etiology. Although good epidemiology is lacking, alcohol, head trauma and multiple sclerosis are probably the most common, although a large number of genetic ataxias are known. The evaluation of ataxia should always include MRI, because computed tomography (CT) does not visualize the posterior fossa well. Acute-onset ataxia suggests a structural lesion (stroke, hemorrhage, trauma) or encephalitis (usually infectious). Subacute ataxia suggests a toxin, neoplasm or a metabolic or some degenerative condition (prion disease), whereas very-slow-onset ataxia suggests a genetic or other neurodegenerative disease.

The treatment of ataxia completely depends on the underlying etiology: surgical excision of tumors or posterior fossa hemorrhages, correction of metabolic conditions, etc. There are no effective treatments for the symptom of ataxia in general. The tremor component may respond to tremor treatments (see Chapter

5) but usually not as well as essential tremor, especially if the tremor is of large amplitude and proximal (oscillating around the shoulder).

Causes of ataxia: differential diagnosis

Focal lesions
Usually posterior fossa (cerebellum and brain stem)
Hemorrhage: immediate neurosurgical intervention required
Tumor
Ischemic stroke
Abscess or any other infectious lesion

Toxic
Ethanol: subacute onset, male predisposition, gait disorder
Phenytoin and (other seizure medications to a lesser extent)
Lithium: acute cerebellar injury with overdose and gradual ataxia with chronic use
Serotonin reuptake inhibitors: part of serotonin syndrome
Radiation therapy: may be delayed by years

Nutritional
Vitamin B_{12} deficiency
Vitamin E deficiency (also genetic causes)
Coenzyme Q10 deficiency (also genetic causes)

Infectious
Herpes encephalitis: often associated with myoclonus
Cerebellaritis: various viral etiologies, CSF diagnosis
Prion disease: CSF 14-3-3 protein and characteristic MRI

Neurodegenerative
Multiple system atrophy – cerebellar (MSA-C): may have parkinsonism
Olivopontocerebellar atrophy: the term is less used as many conditions are now more
    specifically diagnosed; sometimes used interchangeability with MSA-C
Friedreich's ataxia: autosomal recessive, also neuropathy, heart arrhythmias
Ataxia–telangiectasia: childhood onset, conjunctival telangiectasia and susceptibility to
    neoplasm
Many genetic spinal cerebellar ataxias (>30 identified): most autosomal dominant, testing
    available for many of these

Inflammatory/autoimmune
Multiple sclerosis: may have many other neurological manifestations; diagnosis with MRI, CSF
    studies (IgG index and oligoclonal bands) and evoked potentials consistent with
    demyelination
Anti-GAD antibodies (associated with stiff person syndrome)
Acute disseminated encephalitis: acute onset lesions on T2-weighted MRI
Reaction to systemic infection or immunization (rubella, Hemophilus influenzae)

Miscellaneous
Celiac sprue: diagnosis made with antibodies and colon biopsy; responds to gluten-free diet
Paraneoplastic: anti-Yo and anti-Purkinje antibodies; oat cell, ovarian, breast, lymphoma
    cancers
Blunt head trauma: ataxia/tremor onset often delayed and MRI may be normal, usually occurs
    when force is applied to top of head

Figure 6.10 Differential diagnosis of ataxia and comment. CSF, cerebrospinal fluid; GAD, glutamic acid decarboxylase; MRI, magnetic resonance imaging.

Conclusions

The field of movement disorders represents a broad number of phenotypes and most phenotypes include a broad differential diagnosis. In this and the previous chapters we have attempted to classify these by both disease and symptom complex. We estimate that this text covers the diagnosis for more than 95% of all movement disorder patients seen in a specialty clinic. However, an increasing number of rare metabolic conditions, mostly seen in childhood, can present with movement disorders. The most up-to-date summaries for these are usually public genetic databases. In all cases, diagnosis begins with an accurate phenotypic description, which remains the key skill of movement disorder practitioners.

References

1. Correll CU, Schenk EM. Tardive dyskinesia and new antipsychotics. Curr Opin Psychiatry 2008; 21:151–156.
2. Ondo WG, Hanna PA, Jankovic J. Tetrabenazine treatment for tardive dyskinesia: assessment by randomized videotape protocol. Am J Psychiatry 1999; 156:1279–1281.
3. Richardson M, Bevans M, Read L, et al. Efficacy of the branched-chain amino acids in the treatment of tardive dyskinesia in men. Am J Psychiatry 2003; 160:1117-1124.
4. Lerner V, Miodownik C, Kaptsan A, et al. Vitamin B_6 treatment for tardive dyskinesia: a randomized, double-blind, placebo-controlled, crossover study. J Clin Psychiatry 2007; 68: 1648-54
5. Lorberboym M, Treves TA, Melamed E, et al. [^{123}I]–FP/CIT SPECT imaging for distinguishing drug-induced parkinsonism from Parkinson's disease. Mov Disord 2006; 21:510–514.
6. Carroll BT, Lee JW, Graham KT, et al. Diagnosing subtypes of neuroleptic malignant syndrome: an introduction to the Lee–Carroll Scale. Ann Clin Psychiatry 2008; 20:47–48.
7. Boyer E, Shannon M. The serotonin syndrome. N Eng J Med 2005; 352:112-120.
8. Jankovic J. Tourette's syndrome. N Engl J Med 2001; 345:1184–1192.
9. Nakamura K, Aminoff MJ. Huntington's disease: clinical characteristics, pathogenesis and therapies. Drugs Today 2007; 43:97–116.
10. Sitburana O, Ondo WG. Tetrabenazine for hyperglycemic-induced hemichorea–hemiballismus. Mov Disord 2006; 21:2023–2025.

Index